KU-222-874

669 0220105

caring for
older people

SAGE has been part of the global academic community since 1965, supporting high quality research and learning that transforms society and our understanding of individuals, groups and cultures. SAGE is the independent, innovative, natural home for authors, editors and societies who share our commitment and passion for the social sciences.

Find out more at: **www.sagepublications.com**

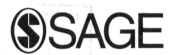

caring for
older people

a shared approach

Christine Brown Wilson

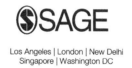

Los Angeles | London | New Delhi
Singapore | Washington DC

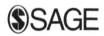

Los Angeles | London | New Delhi
Singapore | Washington DC

SAGE Publications Ltd
1 Oliver's Yard
55 City Road
London EC1Y 1SP

SAGE Publications Inc.
2455 Teller Road
Thousand Oaks, California 91320

SAGE Publications India Pvt Ltd
B 1/I 1 Mohan Cooperative Industrial Area
Mathura Road
New Delhi 110 044

SAGE Publications Asia-Pacific Pte Ltd
3 Church Street
#10-04 Samsung Hub
Singapore 049483

Editor: Susan Worsey
Assistant editor: Emma Milman
Production editor: Katie Forsythe
Copyeditor: Lotika Singha
Proofreader: Sharon Cawood
Marketing manager: Tamara Navaratnam
Cover design: Jennifer Crisp
Typeset by: C&M Digitals (P) Ltd, Chennai, India
Printed by: MPG Books Group, Bodmin, Cornwall

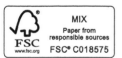

MIX
Paper from
responsible sources
FSC
www.fsc.org   FSC® C018575

Library of Congress Control Number: 2012937456

British Library Cataloguing in Publication data

A catalogue record for this book is available from
the British Library

ISBN 978-1-4462-4096-0
ISBN 978-1-4462-4097-7 (pbk)

To Lesley Wade; my mentor and friend, whose first book on gerontology inspired me to start my journey with older people.

Contents

About the Author

Christine Brown Wilson is a Programme Director in the School of Nursing, Midwifery and Social Work, University of Manchester, United Kingdom. Christine's roles include managing and teaching on a post-registration undergraduate degree programme, research involving older people, including those with dementia, and supporting practice. Christine qualified as a Registered Nurse 30 years ago and has worked with older people in hospital, the community and long-term care. Christine is committed to improving care for older people, including those with dementia through education, research and practice development.

Christine encourages students to use biographical approaches when assessing older people, including those with dementia, and involving older people in care decisions. Christine's initial research focused on relationships between older people, families and staff in long-term care, identifying what approaches to care provide the most positive experience. She has published widely on this subject. Christine is now working with care providers to develop services using these findings. Christine is also health care lead for an interdisciplinary team developing technology to enable older people and those with dementia to remain active in their community. She is particularly interested in how technology supports decision making by health care professionals.

Christine is a member of the National Care Homes Research and Development Forum that provides a network across universities to support collaboration in research and practice development with a view to influencing the policy and research agenda in this area. Christine regularly peer reviews for academic journals and for the National Institute of Health Research Programme.

Foreword

A sea change is occurring in how we think about and what we expect from care homes. Across the world we have seen a growing discontent with the state of affairs in care homes and general recognition that we should expect and need to create something better. Easier said than done! It's not so easy to convert the rhetoric, or even a strong commitment, into the right actions.

Good people with the best of intentions struggle to find ways to create a better space for people who live and work in care homes. Many do not accomplish what they set out to achieve. This leaves people who live in care homes with something less than they deserve (although unfortunately not often less than they expect). It also leaves the committed staff, trying to improve the situation, feeling frustrated. Nothing seems to work.

It's easy to look at care homes we believe are not performing well and villainise the care staff, or the administration or the sector. ... This simply adds to the sense of frustration for staff who have worked so hard and failed to achieve what they know is right. This does not give us a guide for improving things.

So how does Christine Brown Wilson's book fit here? Dr. Brown Wilson has already contributed much to the field, offering us important insights into what really good care might look like. So what does this book add? Dr. Brown Wilson does several important things with this book. Let me start with the care staff. By carefully laying out the various perspectives that used to provide 'really good care', Dr. Brown Wilson allows us all to find ourselves, and to gain insight into both the sources and consequences of the perspective we hold. For some of us this might be uncomfortable, but the discomfort does not come from what Dr. Brown Wilson says about us. It comes from our own insights gained in reading this book. As any effective educator knows, helping someone come to their own insight is much more powerful and lasting than just telling them. Dr. Brown Wilson obviously uses her considerable experience as an educator to walk us up to a place where we can see for ourselves.

She shows us how a particular path, even one often taken by highly committed and well-intentioned care workers, leads us to an end that we would not find satisfactory. She does this without inducing shame or raising questions about the values and motivation of people who find their efforts failing to achieve 'really good care'. This is done gently, in a way that allows the reader to come slowly to a realization without feeling accused. Some readers will find their cherished notions of 'really good care' called into question, by demonstrating where they lead, but they will not feel that their efforts or their motives have been impugned.

Dr. Brown Wilson uses vignettes and activities throughout the book to nudge people to examine where their values, assumptions and perspectives might be leading them. These are subtle but powerful strategies to engage the reader and continuously bring the discussions to a very practical level.

Dr. Brown Wilson weaves the philosophical, empirical and practical together in a way that makes this book quite useful and engaging for researchers, educators and practitioners alike. Being clearly grounded in empirical research, informed throughout by a philosophy of respect for all involved, while offering many practical solutions, is indeed unusual. More often we find one of these three elements alone, leaving us, particularly those in practice, wondering what to do with a particular insight. Dr. Brown Wilson does not stop at insight. She takes us the next step, guiding us in how we might want to put the insight to work. The depth of practical guidance here makes this a very useful resource for people working in and overseeing care homes.

The book is easy to read, engaging, practical and provokes us to reflect on what we are doing, how we are doing it and what we hope to achieve.

Barbara Bowers PhD RN
Helen Denne Schulte Professor
Associate Dean for Research
University of Wisconsin-Madison
School of Nursing

Preface

I have worked with older people in the independent and statutory sectors in the United Kingdom (UK) for the past 25 years. In this time I have seen a very positive trend in seeing older people as individuals, promoting independence and taking into account the needs they identify and choices they make. As a student and newly qualified practitioner, I recognised the importance of care that did not exclusively focus on my professional goals but also incorporated what was important to the older person. Working in the homes of older people enabled me to recognise the importance of independence, inter-dependence and feelings of control for the older person as they experienced a health crisis. We worked together to identify goals that reflected their life aspirations, as well as the professional goals the service needed to provide. I began working in person-centred ways before we had the guidance of recent theoretical models and this experience maintains my enthusiasm and passion for ensuring that we maintain the focus on what is important for older people themselves.

In the present day we are still seeing practice in the UK that falls below the minimum standards we would expect for older people. This is disappointing as much of this substandard practice resonates with findings from some of the early sociological research from the 1960s (Goffman, 1962; Townsend, 1962). Equally, we also know there are areas of very good practice that have improved over the past decade. We are now beginning to see some very positive reports from the care home sector with areas of very good practice (see *My Home Life* [www.myhomelife.org] for examples of this). Unfortunately, this has not been reflected as well in the acute sector with a number of reports outlining very poor care for older people (Abrahams, 2011). That is not to say there is not very good care in the acute sector, but research continues to find pressures of targets impacting on time, resulting in care for older people that often lacks dignity (Brooker et al., 2011; Patterson et al., 2011; Tadd et al., 2011). Areas of positive practice across sectors are often seen when there is leadership, good teamwork and continuity of care (Brown Wilson, 2009; Patterson et al., 2011).

The content within this book draws on research I have undertaken in long term care environments (Brown Wilson, 2009; Brown Wilson and Davies, 2009; Brown Wilson et al., 2009b) incorporating the perspective of older people, families and staff. It became obvious to me as I spent time talking with older people, observing their interactions with each other, their environment and staff supporting them that older people are actively contributing towards their care in ways often not recognised by health and social care staff. Indeed, witnessing the communication style of many nurses, I recognised how we become desensitised to the important information being shared with us as we fail to see the relevance of stories older people share with us. While this might be understandable in the context of the many tasks nurses have to undertake, it means we miss vital information in supporting older people to live meaningful lives, and fulfil their aspirations. Subsequently, I have applied this research to my teaching practice with final year undergraduate nurses and found that many students are witnessing very task-directed practice in both the acute and community environments. However, by using some of the key tenets of my research, many were able to make a real difference to the day-to-day care of older people by being aware of the myths and stereotypes guiding practice with older people, by listening to the stories older people shared with them and then identifying how they might address not only the needs of older people, but also their aspirations. As health and social care practitioners, we do bring professional knowledge and expertise to the relationship when working with older people.

The aim of this book is to provide a means of navigating through the many concepts that have emerged over the past decade related to working with older people, guiding you, the reader, in how these concepts might be put into practice. Although we can see many positive changes in environments caring for older people, there are also times when care for some of the most vulnerable in our society remains sadly lacking. This book provides a supportive approach to working with older people, reminding us of ways of working that sometimes seem so obvious. However, we know that when confronted with a hectic work environment, it is often the most fundamental aspects of working that get forgotten and result in poor or dehumanising approaches to care. This book is not intended to tell you what professional knowledge you need when working with older people – there are many excellent books on evidence-based practice to support you in this. What this book does is provide you with is a way of implementing your professional knowledge using the perspective of the older person, ensuring their goals in life are being met alongside the professional goals practitioners are tasked to deliver. Therefore, this book provides a step-by-step guide in how to work effectively with older people in changing health and social care contexts involving the older person and their families or supporters.

This book seeks to consider how we as practitioners might adjust our practice to consider the needs and aspirations of the older people who need our support as they age. I work on the principle that we change practice one person at a time, starting with ourselves. There are suggestions for how we as individual practitioners might adjust the way we work at different times, enabling us to be more responsive rather than adopting a blanket approach when working with older people. Importantly, we consider how valuing the contribution older people and their families make to their care, might enable nurses in particular to (re)consider their role in bringing the voice of the older person to the decision-making process. This includes ideas for the development of leadership and teamwork that will facilitate teams working in more adaptable and flexible ways, ensuring the needs of older people are being met in ways that involve them in the decision-making process. This will enable us to manage complex care environments, to consider competing needs and still address what is important to the older person and their family.

To achieve this, we need to address some fundamental questions that redirect the focus from ourselves as practitioners to those whom we are supporting:

- How do older people see their health and how does this influence the decisions they make?
- How does what has happened in an older person's life influence their approach to ageing?
- How do we recognise the contribution made by an older person or their carers?
- How might we include older people, families and their supporters in the decision-making process?
- How do we identify what is significant in an older person's life at this point?

  ○ What are the important routines they wish to maintain and how might they be supported in this?
  ○ What are the important relationships in an older person's life and how might the service be impacting on these?

These issues are not unique to this book and as such it should not be read in isolation from other texts that may address each of these issues in more depth. The uniqueness of this book lies in how the student is encouraged to address these issues with the older person as part of their everyday practice.

The case studies throughout this book are derived from both research and practice. The approaches to care were developed from my research in long term care (Brown Wilson, 2007). This work has been published in a number of journals, which I refer to as appropriate throughout the book. There are also previously unpublished examples which are used from this research. Throughout this book I also draw on colleagues' research to demonstrate how the findings from my research in long term care are transferrable to other care environments. The application of many of the principles underpinning the approaches to care developed in my research has been undertaken by undergraduate students as they grapple with applying theory to everyday practice. These examples demonstrate how students have used the underpinning principles within this book to improve the care of older people. To achieve this, these students have valued the perspective of the older person and considered it to have equal merit to the professional perspective. This has meant the student has often had to suspend their professional perspective to hear the voice of the older person and in so doing has then had additional information to inform their professional perspective. The students who have contributed their work throughout this book demonstrate how it is possible to move beyond the immediate needs of the older person to consider their goals and aspirations as well. The examples used within this book all involve real people in real situations, although their identities have been changed, to demonstrate how it is often the simple things that can make a world of difference to an older person, their family and staff. They are designed to encourage you to think differently about the practice situations you find yourself in.

Navigating this book

This book is divided into two parts. Part 1 considers the research that underpins different approaches to care and how recognition of the contribution of older people and their families might improve the experience of care. The chapters are arranged sequentially with an overview of the literature followed by an in-depth exploration of three approaches to care moving from a relatively limited participation with older people and families towards a more participatory approach that involves older people, families and staff in care decisions. The final chapter evaluates the evidence presented in previous chapters to consider how we might integrate the user perspective into quality assessment.

Part 2 considers a range of practical strategies from research and practice that may support staff in adopting the different approaches to care described in the first part of the book. It begins with an outline of some of the popular myths and stereotypes held about older people that student nurses have observed in practice environments. The following chapters are arranged to consider strategies that primarily involve staff towards those that adopt a more participatory approach valuing the contribution of older people, families and staff.

To support you, the reader, in navigating this book, each chapter has a similar format:

- Graded learning outcomes take the student through the description of the content to how to examine and analyse the information, enabling them to develop personal strategies in implementing the information from each chapter.
- Case studies from a range of practice environments show direct application to practice.
- Activities support the student in applying the information within each chapter.
- Final summary of key learning.
- Suggestions for further reading.

The references used throughout this text can be found at the back of the book.

Finally, the term student is used loosely – you may be starting a career in health and social care, returning to study after years of health or social care experience, or involved in continuous professional development, and so there are times when I may use the terms student and practitioner interchangeably. Throughout this book, I consider the student as a developing practitioner, so any learning should then lead to actions as a practitioner. I hope you find this book useful.

Christine Brown Wilson

Acknowledgements

This book would not have been possible without the contribution of older people, families and staff two supported me in my initial research in care homes. They gave their time and insights which provide many of the examples within this book. In my teaching, I often find the concept of successful ageing a difficult one to convey to students. I would like to thank my relative, Marjorie, for her unique insight into how an older person approaches successful ageing. She has proved an inspiration to both me and my students.

Many of the students I teach grapple with the concepts in this book alongside the other demands of their course. In spite of many difficulties, these students have worked hard to apply the principles in sometimes less than understanding environments. I thank them for their contribution to the seminars and sharing their experience which I have tried to capture within this book. You have made a real difference to the lives of older people – you are the future for ensuring these principles become everyday practice – I have great faith in you.

There have also been students who have supported me in communicating some of these principles in ways that have been accessible to their peers, contributing directly to this book. For this I am particularly grateful to: Faye Alexander, Kirsha Anderson, Sarah Bowers, Rachel Brown, Emma Buckley, Chantal Corneill, Dephine Genti, Rhona Johnson, Brenda Kabalira, Thea O'Doherty, Christopher Perry, and Louise Seaward.

This work is based on my PhD for which I acknowledge the supervision and mentorship of Dr Sue Davies and Prof. Mike Nolan. However, the application of these principles across contexts would not have been possible without the support of colleagues who have generously provided me with the findings of their research, in particular Belinda Dewar and Philip Clissett.

I have also been influenced by work undertaken in the USA by Professor Marilyn Rantz and her Quality Improvement Team based at the University of Missouri. I thank them for their welcome and hospitality. The discussions and visits enabled me to understand the US long term care system and how the principles within this book might be applied in the US context.

Last but by no means least, I acknowledge my family – Terry my husband who supports me tirelessly in my work and whose skills in proofreading are invaluable, and my children, Amee and Leigh, who often provide a fresh perspective in our discussions of the issues faced by older people. I would not have been able to complete this book without your love and support, so thank you.

PART 1

UNDERPINNING PRINCIPLES

INTRODUCTION

Working with older people is often seen as something that anyone can do without needing specialist education. This is evidenced in the discipline of nursing by the decline in post-registration qualifications in working with older people and the lack of specialist content in the nursing undergraduate curriculum, particularly in the UK. This book is designed to provide students with an evidence-based framework that will support them to articulate their contribution when working with older people in an inter-disciplinary context. I have spoken to university educators in the USA, Australia and Canada, where everyone shared common stories about the difficulties in promoting the older person in the nursing curriculum. This may be because working with older people remains undervalued both by curriculum managers as well as by students themselves. This book provides practical strategies to support students and educators to articulate what makes working with older people so important and rewarding.

THE DEMOGRAPHICS: WHAT ARE THE IMPLICATIONS FOR HEALTH AND SOCIAL CARE?

We are living in an ageing society where older people are beginning to out-number younger people in many countries in the developing world (World Health Organization [WHO], 2009). Asian countries have a high proportion of older people, with Japan having the 'oldest' population in the developed world. Although previously many Asian countries could depend on families for providing care and support, this is becoming less common (Lee and Mason, 2011). In Western developed countries, we are beginning to see the generation commonly known as 'baby boomers', who were born in the post-war years to the early 1960s, now entering their later life. These people have come through a highly consumerist culture and have differing expectations of services. This means the current 'low-level' expectations that older people hold of health and social care (Tadd et al., 2011) are likely to change with successive waves of the baby boomer generation.

We are also seeing a growing global trend where the birth rate is falling below replacement level in many countries (Lee and Mason, 2011). In the UK, for example, fewer babies are being born compared with the numbers of people who are dying (Baylis and Sly, 2010), which means that in coming years there will be fewer people working to pay the taxes that currently fund state support for older people in retirement. This will have future implications for the National Health Service (NHS) if care is to remain free at the point of delivery. This is a growing phenomenon across the world as many governments consider the financial implications of supporting a growing population of older people.

Older people are also living longer in retirement than in the years they had been working. Although longevity is currently increasing (i.e. the length of time older people are living for), many of these years are spent with disability, primarily due to life-limiting chronic conditions, which may account for the higher numbers of people aged 60 and over using health care services (Dew, 2011). With the growing population of older people, healthcare utilisation remains an area for concern as older people tend to be treated in emergency departments as unscheduled admissions more frequently for conditions that could be treated in less acute environments (Gruneir et al., 2011). Part of the reason for this may be that there are insufficient community-based services available to support older people in managing their health more effectively. If the additional years many older people are living are to be disability-free, there needs to be a greater emphasis on promoting health and activity for this group as long as possible.

THE PATIENT JOURNEY: DOES CONTEXT MATTER?

We are now seeing an ongoing squeeze on resources with policy focusing on keeping older people living in their community for as long as possible. This is partly due to the increased cost of residential environments, and partly because this is what older people choose. The focus on health and social care policy has and will continue to be on promoting independence, autonomy and choice, enabling older people to live in their community for longer (WHO, 2002). This is reflected in different government initiatives such as the monitoring of the discharge of older people from hospital to ensure they return sooner to a community environment for intermediate care or re-enablement services. One such indicator being used is how many people are still living at home three months after their discharge from hospital and this figure is currently at 78% for England (NHS Information, 2012).

Although older people wish to stay in their homes for longer, in the English Longitudinal Study into Ageing (ELSA) wellbeing scores were found to decrease after age 65. This suggested that as people age, their wellbeing reduces in the control they feel they have over their environment; the opportunities they have to make decisions without unwanted interference; and their sense of fulfilment or pleasure derived from the more active aspects of life. This decrease in wellbeing may be attributed to factors such as poorer health in later life, loss of immediate family or friends and reduced mobility in older age (Baylis and Sly, 2010). However, if we are supporting a growing population of older people who are living longer, possibly with life-limiting conditions, we need to (re)consider how we conceptualise health and social care to improve the quality of life for older people through the services we provide.

While nursing espouses a 'holistic approach', many students I teach continue to raise concerns about the lack of time available to consider the needs of older people. This is compounded by the focus on tasks so that when students are speaking with older people, they feel they should be 'doing' something else. Many of the stories student nurses recount include small acts that take little time but make a real difference to the wellbeing of the older person. This suggests that time spent in conversation with the older person may be transferred effectively into their care, even in the busiest environments. To value time spent in conversation, we need to see the older person not just as a recipient of care but a person capable of self-fulfilment and pleasure derived from the more active aspects of life.

This book is divided into two parts. Part 1 outlines the underpinning principles of approaches to care derived initially from research I have undertaken in long-term care. The discussion is underpinned by student examples of how they have applied these principles in other contexts. Part 2 provides practical examples from research and practice to demonstrate how these approaches might be enacted across different care environments to support older people more effectively.

Part 1 presents three approaches to care that focus on relationships in different ways. Each approach involves the older person, their family and staff, and is broken down into easily identifiable components that can be integrated into everyday health and social care practice. The final chapter in Part 1 considers how we might use this information to reconceptualise quality, given the policy debates on the 'user experience'.

Chapter 1 critically examines the notion of patient-centred, person-centred and relationship-centred care from a policy and practice perspective. The chapter discusses what each of these terms means in practice and how they might be operationalised to enhance the experience of the older person.

Chapter 2 presents the individualised task-centred approach to care. This approach supports preferences for older people, knowing what they like to eat and when they like to get up/go to bed, etc. This approach infers good quality clinical care that focuses solely on physical aspects of caregiving. Individualising care in this way can support staff in avoiding poor clinical care.

Chapter 3 discusses how a person-centred approach promotes understanding of why something is significant in an older person's life. This moves beyond likes and dislikes to understanding why different routines or aspects of a person's care are important to them by locating this information in the context of a person's biography. The chapter focuses on the contribution older people and families make to supporting the development of this knowledge through the stories people share.

Chapter 4 presents a way of considering the organisational context of care, enabling person-centred care to be delivered in a busy communal context. The relationship-centred approach is presented so that the needs of everyone involved in the relationship – older people, families and staff – might be considered.

Chapter 5 considers the impact that the different approaches discussed in the preceding chapters might have on older people, families and staff, and how this might influence what is meant by a 'quality service'. An alternative approach to quality is proposed that reflects the experience of older people and their families by considering how the quality of care might be assessed using the following concepts: care that satisfies 'me'; care that matters to 'me'; care that involves 'all of us'.

CHAPTER 1

Defining the continuum of care for older people

Learning outcomes

After reading this chapter, the student will be able to:

- Identify the key attributes of person-centred care
- Describe how person-centred care might differ from other approaches of care
- Describe what is meant by relationship-centred care
- Critically examine the differences between the different approaches along a continuum of care that seek to integrate the perspective of staff, older people and their families

Introduction

Within the literature there is a range of terms that are at times used interchangeably within practice, but do not always mean the same thing. This contributes to confusion within the practice environment as to which approach is best adopted and how such approaches might be incorporated into everyday practice. This may result in nurses reverting back to an approach to practice where they know the job will get done. Lack of time and other organisational constraints beyond their control are often given as reasons why nurses are unable to do more than focus on the task (Bradbury-Jones et al., 2011). Student nurses also struggle to focus on the person as they contend with the range of environments, the different approaches to mentorship with older people and the pressure of their university assessments (Brown et al., 2008).

Different ways of conceptualising care in relation to the individuality of people emerged within the 1990s as a more consumerist approach to health care was being adopted both in the UK, United States (US) and Australia. In considering the literature of the 1990s in respect to developing relationships, a number of models emerged from a very functional approach to patient-centred (Lutz and Bowers, 2000) and person-centred care to approaches that valued the personhood of the older person (Kitwood, 1997). Relationship-centred care also emerged to consider the wider relationships within the community and how this influenced the person's approach to their health (Tresolini and the Pew-Fetzer Task Force, 1994). In reviewing these different approaches, we see a pattern of movement from health care being 'done to a person' to becoming an increasingly 'shared' endeavour. This chapter presents a systematic synthesis of this literature.

This chapter presents a synthesis of the literature, based on concept analysis (Risjord, 2009). Published literature, including grey literature such as doctorial theses, was searched to identify the key models of person-centred, patient-centred and relationship-centred care. One of the key themes that spanned these models was the concept of participation. I considered how central the concept of participation was to each model and the stakeholders that this participation extended to. These stakeholders could include older people, families, or staff.

Undertaking a concept analysis such as this has its limitations. For example, much of the literature is theoretical with limited empirical research available within this field. This means that it may be difficult to generalise findings. In addition, this analysis is subjective, based on my personal interpretation of what participation might mean within each of these models. However, this analysis provides a staring point by which we might consider what participation might mean from the perspective of older people, families and staff in different contexts of care.

In previous work I have undertaken (Brown Wilson and Davies, 2009), the approach staff adopted often influenced the ability of the older person or family member to be involved in care. Therefore, I have used the following approaches of staff to discuss the synthesis of the literature in relation to participation:

- Seeing the task
- Seeing the person
- Seeing the relationships

In addition to discussing the synthesis of the literature, I will be using case studies that demonstrate the end result of adopting each of these different themes.

Seeing the task

Wherever we are supporting older people, when our main focus is on the task, we adopt an attitude towards the older person which is then communicated in ways that we often don't recognise.

Practice scenario: Medical unit

Martha was admitted with a chest infection. During the assessment Martha mentions activities that she has been struggling with at home. The priority for the nurse was that Martha's chest infection was treated and so she told Martha that everything else would be dealt with later. Martha was prescribed antibiotics and intravenous fluids for dehydration with her fluid balance monitored. These activities were focused on the restoration of health and very necessary. However, Martha was made to feel that the other issues she had concerns about were not important to the nurse. This would make it difficult for Martha to tell the nurse what was on her mind in future.

We might be concerned about the time needed to work with an older person given the pressures of our workload. This means there may be a tendency to label all older people as 'hard work', or even 'nuisances'. When older people enter the acute setting, they initially ignore assaults on their dignity that come from these attitudes (Jacelon, 2003). Labels can also be created to help us categorise people and may even be used as a form of shorthand. For example, as professionals, we tend to label older people according to the services they are receiving; this may be as patients in health care, clients in community care, service users or residents in long-term care. If we take the example of the label 'patients', this denotes the fact that someone has entered an acute hospital setting and professionals expect people to have the attributes of a 'patient' – requiring support from registered professionals who have the knowledge and skills to help that person, often in an acute crisis. However, many older people do not fit the 'neat package' that the label 'patient' infers and many nurses struggle to provide the care required for older people with complex needs. Jacelon (2003) found that as older people move into the recovery phase, they begin to feel out of context and disrespected by staff. To address this, older people tend to adopt interactive strategies to manage their image and establish reciprocal relationships. If staff do not recognise these actions or consider such actions to be time-consuming, it then becomes more difficult for older people to engage fully in the consultative process within a hospital setting.

Older people are labelled in wider society as well; by referring to them as 'the elderly', for example, older people are placed in a homogeneous group that is somehow 'different'. This means that when we make decisions about the care of an older person, we begin to rationalise that this is okay, because they are this 'group' of people who require a certain 'type' of care. From this starting point, it isn't that far to rationalise poor care because there are other more pressing priorities. This is reminiscent of the term 'task-centred' used by nurse researchers in the 1970s and 1980 to define care that was dictated by the organisation. The term task-centred became synonymous with care that did not take into account the needs expressed by older people as nurses tended to see their work as a collection of tasks to be undertaken, forgetting that they were dealing with a person. To see the role of nursing as a collection of tasks then places older people at an immediate disadvantage as nurses often perceive older people as a group of people who require more time and may therefore be relegated down a priority list. Tadd et al. (2011), for example, describe how newly qualified nurses in one acute hospital spoke about the difficulties of managing care to ensure older people received even the most fundamental care due to increasing pressures at ward level. Therefore, to say that care focusing on the task no longer exists would be naïve, particularly when faced with competing priorities in a busy clinical environment.

It could be argued that focusing on the task ensures older people receive good-quality clinical care but putting the needs of the organisation above the needs of the older person often results in poor clinical care (Abrahams, 2011). To balance competing priorities, such as when an older person is acutely ill or when there are staff shortages, we need to consider how we might focus on the task and ensure individualised care at the same time. This approach ensures clinical needs are met taking into account the preference and choice of an older person and will be discussed in more detail in Chapter 2.

ACTIVITY

Identifying the key priorities

Choose an example from your experience in practice where an older person was asked to wait for care due to prioritisation of 'other' tasks such as a medication round. Write brief answers to the following:

- What were the key factors in the decision to prioritise the 'other' task?
- What were your concerns had you not prioritised the 'other' task?
- What was the impact on the older person?

Keep these answers, as we will use this example as we progress through the remainder of this chapter to consider different strategies that might be available to inform how you manage similar situations in future.

Health care reform and policy initiatives focused on improving the quality of care for older people now encourage professionals to take into account the needs and preferences expressed by older people. When older people are perceived as a homogeneous group, this means we give all older people the same characteristics, which might prevent us from seeing each older person as an individual. Student nurses in particular find it hard to develop a focus on the older person depending on the clinical environment in which they work. Once students feel their course objectives will be met in practice, they are then more able to focus on the patient (Brown et al., 2008). It is for this reason we need to consider how different approaches to care might support us in seeing patients as individuals in their own right, not as a group of people.

Seeing the person

Patient-centred care as a term seems to be medically based, aimed at supporting medical professionals to see the person beyond the patient. The Institute of Medicine (IOM), for example, has included patient-centred care as a criterion for improving health care quality in the USA. The definition of patient-centred care from the IOM suggests practitioners should be responsive to needs, values and expressed preferences, show compassion and empathy, provide for physical comfort and emotional support, relieve fear and anxiety, and involve family and friends. Other aspects include: co-ordination and integration, providing information, communicating effectively and patient education (IOM, 2001). Goodrich and Cornwell (2008) conducted a research project in the UK acute sector and found that professionals could not describe all of the dimensions of patient-centred care even in their own words. They often spoke about *attitudes* aimed at improving patient care or *actions* specifically associated with protecting patients' privacy and dignity. A key limitation of the IOM definition is the exclusive focus on the immediate context. It does not take into account the importance of a person's life beyond their current experience of health or illness.

In a conceptual analysis of the term 'patient-centred care', Lutz and Bowers defined this concept as 'identifying patients' needs, preferences and expectations and re-organising health services to meet patients' needs' (2000: 177). This is not dissimilar to the IOM definition in that the focus is on the immediate needs for services. Similarly, the term 'person-centred care' used in UK government policies defines a more service-oriented approach: taking into account the person's needs over the needs of the service (Department of Health [DH], 2000). The definition of person-centred care in UK policy is focused on the creation of services that meet the needs of individual people, based on the person's need rather than the requirements of the service. While this is to be welcomed, the definition remains functional; by this I mean the focus is primarily on the task required. These definitions support us in redefining services to consider the importance of choice but make it difficult to move beyond the task as there remains limited recognition of the importance of participation for older people. This is in direct contrast to the concept of patient-centred care as described in a community context. Mead and Bower (2000) suggest patient-centred care includes the sharing of power and responsibility between the medical practitioner and patient, taking into account social and psychological (as well as biomedical) factors; developing common therapeutic goals that understand the personal meaning of the illness for each individual. These different definitions of patient-centred care suggest that different contexts may require different approaches to care.

The term 'patient-centred care' reflects the medical context of definitions we have discussed so far. Alternatively, the term 'person-centred care' suggests a more sociological approach, whereby it is the person who is the focus rather than the medical condition or context of the care encounter. The term person-centred care was initially used within dementia care to encourage staff to respect the personhood of the person with dementia, recognising their need for inclusion, attachment, comfort, identity and occupation (Kitwood, 1997). Kitwood suggested that 'malignant social psychology' enacted by staff and influenced by the environment often robbed people with dementia of their self-esteem and confidence. Subsequently, Brooker (2004) developed the VIPS model of person-centred care to provide a clearer direction in developing person-centred care: Value of all human lives; Individualised approach recognising uniqueness; seeing the world from the Perspective of the service user; Social environment that promotes wellbeing. This model is designed to support staff in engaging with the person with dementia as a person first, to consider what is important to them. Relationships with others are implicit in this model with the key focus being on the staff and person with dementia.

Practice scenario: Medical unit

Mrs Fletcher was admitted with a diagnosis of dementia. She appeared quite agitated and aggressive, which led staff to avoid her. The student spent time listening to Mrs Fletcher's concerns, which showed she was valued. Having previously been a teacher, there were times Mrs Fletcher thought she was back in the schoolroom, controlling unruly children, which explained her behaviour. This information helped staff understand Mrs Fletcher's perspective , which led to more individualised care.

In a review of the literature, McCormack (2004) described the key themes within models of person-centred practice as:

- Knowing the person and how they see their illness
- The importance of values of the person and staff member working with them
- The biography of the person
- Relationships with significant others as well as the staff working with them
- Staff being able to see beyond the immediate needs of the older person

McCormack and McCance (2006) suggest a model for person-centred practice that considers how the attitudes of the nurse and context of care influence the processes of person-centred care. The nurse recognising their own beliefs and values as well as the beliefs and values of the older person is central to this model. Working with older people in this way is not easy to define. McCormack and McCance (2010) suggest a person-centred nursing framework using the following components:

- The attributes of the nurse such as competence, awareness of personal beliefs and values

- The care environment such as the skill mix, the physical environment or the organisation of care
- person-centred processes such as working with patients' beliefs and values and shared decision making
- person-centred outcomes, such as the older person's involvement with care or feeling of wellbeing

Both of the person-centred models we have reviewed so far consider the centrality of the personhood of the older person with a focus on the interaction between the staff and the older person. The role of the older person in both of these models remains implicit, which means there is limited guidance on how we might achieve person-centred processes. One of the key shortcomings of the models presented so far is the lack of recognition of the combined contribution of older people, families and staff.

My research in long-term care suggests that older people and their families also make a contribution to the relationships that develop (Brown Wilson et al., 2009b). A key feature of seeing the person is knowing what is important to that person through the significant details in their life, such as routines they enjoy, activities which hold meaning in their lives or the importance of wearing jewellery or makeup. This information is actively shared by older people and their families, and for person-centred care to be enacted, the contribution older people and families make also needs to be valued and acted upon. This will be considered in more detail in Chapter 3.

Reviewing the key priorities

Refer back to your example from practice where an older person was asked to wait for care due to prioritisation of 'other' tasks. Now consider the following:

- What belief or values influenced your decision to prioritise the 'other' task?
- What aspects of the care environment contributed to your decision to prioritise the 'other' task?
- How important was the care routine for the older person?
- How might you have involved the older person in this decision?

Keep these answers, as we will continue with this example as we progress through the remainder of this chapter.

ACTIVITY

While the importance of relationships is implicit within the person-centred models described above, the focus remains on how relationships impact on the wellbeing of the older person. Arguably, this carries a risk of not considering the issues of other stakeholders involved in caring for older people. Alternatively, Nolan et al. (2004) suggest that it is not only the personhood of the older person that needs to be considered, but also the personhood of staff and family caregivers, and that relationship-centred care enables this to be achieved.

Seeing the relationship

Relationships are central to the care-giving process (Brown Wilson et al., 2009b) and relationship-centred care recognises that relationships are central to the therapeutic encounter (Tresolini and the Pew-Fetzer Task Force, 1994). Relationship-centred care goes beyond the exclusive focus on the doctor–patient relationship as outlined in patient-centred care, to consider relationships between other practitioners as well as between the person and their community. This model was intended to support the education of medical community practitioners based in the USA, helping them to see beyond the physical needs of the patient. Relationship-centred care is based on a therapeutic relationship which should have as its foundation a shared understanding of what health and illness mean to the person and those close to them, in the context of the community in which they live (Beach et al., 2006). However, it goes beyond the holistic person-centred model to include an appreciation of the whole person, recognition of the person's life story and the impact of the community in which they live (Tresolini and the Pew-Fetzer Task Force, 1994). To achieve relationship-centred care, practitioners need to possess the following skills, knowledge and values to build therapeutic relationships:

- Self-awareness and the ability to reflect on one's own practice
- Understanding of what life in the community means to the (older) person
- The ability to develop relationships (with the older person)
- The ability to work as a team
- The ability to work with practitioners across organisations

Relationship-centred care has been further developed within a UK context to reflect the perspective (and needs) of family caregivers and staff alongside the perspective (and needs) of the older person, creating a more participatory approach. Nolan et al. suggest that relationship-centred care is enacted when the six Senses (security, significance, continuity, belonging, purpose, achievement) are experienced by older people, their families and staff:

> the Senses Framework captures the important dimensions of interdependent relationships necessary to create and sustain an enriched environment of care in which all participants are acknowledged and addressed. This lies at the heart of our vision of relationship centred care and illustrates the delicate interactions necessary to achieve truly collaborative care. (2006: 124)

There is growing empirical evidence for the Senses Framework in a range of care environments, including acute services (Patterson et al., 2011), dementia care (Ryan et al., 2008; Brown Wilson et al., 2012) and community services (Clissett and Brown Wilson, in press). Each of 'the Senses' are subjective, which means they may be enacted in different ways, making the Senses Framework difficult to assess across contexts. For example, some Senses might be actively created, whereas others might spontaneously occur and this may be different across contexts.

Practice scenario: Medical unit

Mrs Buck had been previously independent at home but during her hospital stay became unhappy. Having a very active lifestyle normally, Mrs Buck told the student how she was beginning to lose her sense of purpose in life. Mrs Buck was encouraged to go to the hospital shop each morning and she would ask each of the other women in her bay if they wanted anything. This gave Mrs Buck a sense of purpose, belonging and achievement as she regained her independence.

Relationships are also central to the experience of older people and their families in acute care. In a meta-synthesis of the literature, Bridges et al. (2010) found that good and bad aspects of care were described in relational terms. Three key themes emerged as: maintaining identity (see who I am); shared decision making (involve me) and creating communities (connect with me). Dewar (2011) suggests that compassionate conversations enable staff to know what matters to the person and then to work with that person to shape the way things are done, thus achieving compassionate relationship care. These features resonate with relationship-centred care as conceptualised by Nolan et al. (2006). However, in my research, it was recognised that older people, families and staff may hold differing perspectives, therefore, to achieve relationship-centred care, an element of negotiation and compromise may be required to ensure the needs of everyone in the relationship are taken into account. My research suggests that staff engage in negotiation and compromise with each other, with older people and families to enable everyone to contribute as part of the community and this forms an important feature in relationship-centred care (Brown Wilson et al., 2009b). This will be discussed in more detail in Chapter 4.

Developing our priorities to provide relationship-centred care

ACTIVITY

Refer back to your example from practice where an older person was asked to wait for care due to prioritisation of 'other' tasks. Now consider the following:

- How might you have involved other members of the multi-disciplinary team to meet the needs of the older person?

(Continued)

(Continued)

- How might you involve an older person in decision making at times when you do not need to prioritise tasks in this way?
- How might care be organised to support the care of older people more effectively?

The answers from each of the activities within this chapter provide you with a starting point from which you might consider how to improve the care of older people within your context of care. We will be considering a range of underpinning principles and practical strategies throughout this book to support you in developing your practice further.

When I was undertaking my research, I observed staff in the same care environment adopting different approaches to practice at different times of the day. Hughes et al. (2008) suggest that there are similar themes within concepts such as person-centred or relationship-centred care and that the interaction with the person, in different contexts, might require a different approach by health care professionals. For example, a one-to-one encounter with an older person might require a person-centred approach, whereas working with a group of people might require a relationship-centred approach in order to meet the needs of everyone in the relationship. My own experience as an individual practitioner suggests that it is possible to engage in a person-centred approach, but this lacks consistency when you are not on duty. To ensure a more consistent approach for person-centred care, we need to adopt different ways of working; this may involve negotiation and compromise which move us towards a more participatory way of working as identified in a relationship-centred approach to care.

Summary

- Older people are not a homogeneous group and will require an individualised approach to care.
- Terms such as patient-centred and person-centred care are not necessarily synonymous and need to be critically evaluated according to the context of care.
- Person-centred care moves beyond individualised preferences and choice to consider how a person's biography might shape their care.
- Relationship-centred care focuses on the positive relationships that exist between older people, families and staff moving towards a more participatory approach to care where all perspectives are valued.
- Different contexts might require different approaches to care.

Conclusion

In this chapter we have discussed different models of patient-centred, person-centred and relationship-centred care. These models articulate involving the older person and practitioner in different ways, such as encouraging the development of shared goals or shared decision making compared with ensuring services fulfil the needs of individuals. Some models also involve others beyond the person–caregiver dyad to include family, other professionals and the community. This suggests that different models encourage different levels of participation by the older person, their family and staff. Older people are not a homogeneous group and so may need different approaches, involving different people, sometimes within the same environment of care. It is important to appreciate that staff bring their own values, beliefs and attitudes when supporting older people, which may also influence the approach adopted. Therefore, a 'one size fits all' mentality might not be the best way of improving care of the older person. We will explore how we might develop a more flexible approach to caring for older people in subsequent chapters.

Further reading

Brown, J., Robb, Y., Lowndes, A., Duffy, K., Tolson, D. and Nolan, M. (2011) 'Understanding relationships within care', in Tolson, D., Booth, J. and Schofield, I. (eds), *Evidence Informed Nursing with Older People*. Oxford: Wiley Blackwell.

Clarke, C. (2011) 'Fundamentals in nursing', in Reed, J., Clarke, C. and McFarlane, A. (eds), *Nursing Older People: A Textbook for Nurses*. Buckinghamshire: Open University Press.

McCormack, B. and McCance, T. (2010) *Person Centred Nursing: Theory and Practice.* Oxford: Wiley Blackwell.

Reed, J. and McCormack, B. (2011) 'Independence and autonomy, the foundation of care', in Reed, J., Clarke, C. and McFarlane, A. (eds), *Nursing Older People: A Textbook for Nurses*. Buckinghamshire: Open University Press.

CHAPTER 2

Focusing on the task

Learning outcomes

By the end of this the chapter, the reader will be able to:

- Describe how care routines might be individualised by getting to know the older person
- Develop strategies that might promote an individualised task-centred approach to care
- Critically examine how motivation to care might impact on how staff approach their care
- Consider how the contribution of older people and their supporters might influence the care process

Introduction

All nurses are facing increasing pressure to focus on service delivery outcomes, much of which emphasise efficiency and professional definitions of effectiveness. This seems to be moving nursing towards a continued focus on achieving measurable tasks, which might initially seem to be in direct contrast to the experience of older people and their families, who often describe good or bad care in terms of relationships (Bridges et al., 2010). In my research, I often observed staff using care routines as a mechanism to get to know the needs and preferences of the older person. On these occasions, staff were able to find out the person's preferences and choices and were able to individualise care, but they remained focused on the task of caregiving. This can best be described as individualised task-centred care (Figure 2.1). Staff, who described their motivation as 'doing a good job', described an individualised task-centred approach to care. For these staff, care centred on ensuring the tasks were done, but in a way that recognised the individuality of the older person. This was often in environments that were physically and emotionally demanding. Often the bottom line for older people and their supporters is that they receive good clinical care and there may be times when this is only possible if an individualised task-centred approach is adopted. New staff, for example, might begin with this approach as they get to know people's individual routines as well as the organisational routines within which they operate. For staff with cultural backgrounds different from the older people they care for, an individualised task approach becomes a good starting point to understand the different cultural expectations of long-term care in the UK. There may also be times when older people feel unwell or experience a health crisis and simply want good clinical care until they feel able to resume the usual pattern of their life. An individualised task-centred approach infers good quality clinical care that focuses on physical aspects of care while recognising the individual preferences of the older person.

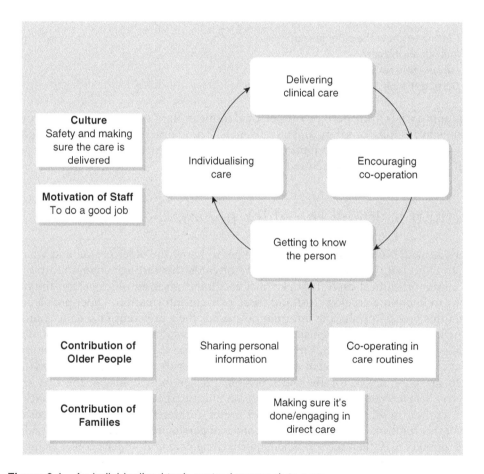

Figure 2.1   An individualised task-centred approach to care

In Chapter 1 we saw how the different conceptualisations of care have moved our professional thinking towards favouring the individualisation of care for older people. While this respects the choice and preferences of older people, encouraging their independence, it has become confused with person-centred care. Many people are now adopting an individualised task-centred approach in their organisations, which is to be welcomed, but the focus remains on the task of care rather than the person. This is not to say older people receiving this approach do not receive good clinical care but it might be described as inconsistent as other priorities might be considered to be more important to 'get the job done'. It may be that staff feel they have no option but to focus on the task but then don't realise that providing individualised care is not necessarily being person-centred. This chapter will support you in identifying when individualised task-centred care is occurring in your area of clinical practice. The key processes which support an individualised task-centred approach include:

- Getting to know the older person
- Individualising care
- Encouraging co-operation
- Getting the job done

This approach is influenced by the personal motivation of staff to do a good job and a dominant culture of safety and effectiveness. The chapter concludes by looking at how recognition of the contribution of older people and their families might support staff in adopting a person-centred approach to care.

Getting to know the older person

Working with older people requires us to get to know the older person and what it is they expect of the clinical encounter. We often do this through communication as we engage in clinical care. This personal encounter gives an older person the time to get to know us, develop trust and share relevant information. Older people may begin this process by sharing information such as their preference for daily routines in personal hygiene. Recognising that an older person has left their meal might prompt a conversation about meal preferences where they provide information on what food they like or at what times they may prefer to eat. This approach enables us to promote choice for the older person, further individualising the care they receive. When older people are able to communicate, they may provide feedback to care workers in what they like or if they prefer a different approach. When recognised, this feedback begins to develop a store of personal knowledge that individual care workers may then rely on when approaching care with older people, changing their approach to reflect the individual requirements of the older person. The detail in achieving this might not always be recorded as it is considered the usual approach to their practice. Alternatively, when older people are not able to communicate verbally, such as following a stroke or when living with dementia, the process of getting to know someone may occur through trial and error as demonstrated in the following practice scenario.

> ## Practice scenario: Care homes (Brown Wilson, 2007)
>
> Many older people have conditions such as stroke or dementia that cause issues with verbal communication. Understanding a person's usual routine was one way staff in care homes managed these communication difficulties. For example, one staff member described how she would use the circumstances in which someone was communicating – if the person was in the dining room, they might want another drink or not like what they were eating. If the person was used to having a rest in the afternoon, then communication may be related to that. However, there were times when it was a bit of trial and error to make sure the staff member knew what was wrong.

Individualised care has a strong tradition in nursing as a means of humanising care and increasing job satisfaction of nurses. It is also seen as an antidote to the inflexibility of organisational routines. Taking into account an older person's expressed needs or preferences is central to individualising care routines but as such it tends to focus care on the practical nature of the caregiving task. This focus on the practical nature of care giving may often stifle opportunities for social conversation as the focus remains on the practical tasks being undertaken.

Creating an individualised routine of care

We all have routines in our daily lives. It might be in how we get up in the morning; whether we shower or have a wash, when we have a cup of tea or coffee and how that makes us feel. We all know that when our usual routine is interrupted, our day often gets off to a bad start. Equally there are times when we value a change to our usual routine, a degree of flexibility in how we might approach our day. The difference between ourselves and an older person in a hospital or care environment is that we control our start to the day while the older person has limited control over their day.

'Routine' has become a much demonised term within the literature, representing care that favours the organisation over the individual (Brown Wilson et al., 2009b). In a concept analysis, Zisberg et al. propose the definition of routine as:

> a concept pertaining to strategically designed behaviour patterns (conscious and subconscious) used to organise and co-ordinate activities along the axes of time, duration, social and physical contexts, sequence and order. (2007: 446)

Older people I have spoken to in a number of care environments describe the routines of the day as markers providing structure and organisation. However, we must also recognise that the need for structure is not uniform; it may be personality driven or reflect an individual's lifestyle. For older people with declining cognitive abilities, the structure of the day and routines they recognise become very important to them. From a staff perspective, routines enable staff to ensure everyone receives the care they need and allow efficient allocation of resources when these are limited (Zisberg et al., 2007).

Developing an individualised plan of care

Draw a table with three columns:

- In the first column, list the ways you get to know an older person
- In the second column, list the type of information shared with you
- In the third column, list how you might individualise routines of care

Delivering clinical care

In my research, practice and teaching experience I have never yet come across an older person or family member who was happy with poor clinical care. Individualised task-centred care is a mechanism that can support staff in improving clinical care while getting to know the older person's preferences on a practical level. This will support staff in achieving the practical tasks that are required such as ambulation and toileting, which can then be seen as a visible marker of quality (Rantz and Zwygart-Stauffacher, 2004). Some older people wish to receive good technical care and not move into relationships beyond this (Bowers et al., 2001a).

All health and social care contexts have an organisational routine and when you are caring for many people, often the organisational routines need to be considered, although in an individualised task-centred approach, they are not the main focus of care. However, to ensure we can provide good clinical care for everyone, we often need older people to co-operate in their care. Promoting independence is an appropriate way to encourage co-operation – the expectation that older people will do things for themselves is a central tenet of what older people say they want. Enabling older people to do things for themselves in their personal care routines is often a good way of demonstrating how you are promoting independence.

However, there are limitations to an exclusive focus on the practical nature of delivering clinical care as this focus tends to limit the opportunities for conversation and therefore limit the exchange of personal information.

In personal care routines, for example, we may focus on gaining the co-operation of the resident to promote independence, but in a way that enables us to complete our workload. We must also recognise that this approach communicates to older people that nurses only have limited time and so would not be interested in more personal information they may wish to share. I observed this most clearly in the focus of interactions between staff and older people in the early morning routines in care homes, with a similar pattern being reported in more acute environments (Wadensten, 2005). The content of morning time conversations, chosen by staff, often sets the tone of the day, influencing the nature of social interactions and so the information being shared by the older person.

Clinical assessment also needs to be conducted in ways that demonstrate we recognise an individual's needs and preferences. The assessment procedures used in health and social care environments consider the key activities of daily living adopting a risk management approach. We undertake these assessments through a professional lens using the language we are most familiar with. In the case of health care, we adopt a more medicalised view of risk as opposed to social care, which will adopt a more personalised view of risk. In both arenas, when caring for an older person, we routinely undertake an assessment and then formulate a plan of care.

In long-term care environments, the care plan will be discussed with the older person who sign the document when able. Families may also be involved in these discussions, being asked to sign the documents when an older person is not able to do so. There may be times when professionals working in health care environments will formulate a care plan based on information provided by the older person, their supporters and other records but they may not always share this plan of care with the older person. This might be appropriate at times when an older person is acutely ill, but is not necessarily appropriate as the person is recovering and moving to a rehabilitative phase. Involving the older person in reviewing documentation is the first step towards ensuring that individualised care is achieved alongside an appropriate level of recording.

Practice scenario: Community

Mrs Smith is an 82-year-old woman who was spending most of her days in bed due to pain. She was a new patient to the caseload of a district nurse whom a student was accompanying. The district nurse explained that the purpose of the visit was to make a an assessment of needs for the new patient. The student realised that they had already made an assessment – before they had sat down and spoken to Mrs Smith, with the clinical judgement that Mrs Smith's main problem was the management of pain so she could mobilise around the house. On subsequent visits, the student began speaking to Mrs Smith who confided that her main priority would be to resume outings to the village with her husband.

Individualised task-centred care is often the easiest way to demonstrate we are delivering good quality clinical care, as we can record measurable clinical outcomes. From the previous practice scenario, we can see that this approach might not always focus on what is significant or meaningful for the older person. Individualised task-centred care may also recognise the contribution of families and older people in the completion of paperwork such as social histories. Activities such as these provide a record of how we have involved both older people and families, which is considered good practice. However, to achieve good clinical care across shifts, a number of factors need to be considered, including the personal motivation of staff as well as leadership and teamwork.

Personal motivation of staff: 'doing a good job'

We all enter caring professions for different reasons and at different points in our lives. We may have had experience of caring for relatives or friends, which gave us an interest in becoming involved in nursing or it might have been a lifetime ambition which we are now in a position to realise. We might not have even meant to end up working with older people, but now find ourselves in this position. Within my research, staff described a personal motivation of 'doing a good job' as the reason they were in care work and described this as undertaking the tasks of caring to the best of their abilities, which they believed had positive consequences for the older people they cared for (Brown Wilson, 2009).

'Doing a good job' in my research was described as a personal philosophy by care workers, which gave them a sense of pride in 'a job well done' by delivering good clinical care while still respecting the individuality of older people. This has also been noted in other studies on acute wards with staff describing 'a good job' as making sure someone had their bed changed even though it was five minutes before they went home because it was the right thing to do (Dewar, 2011). In a study with health care workers in acute dementia wards, Schneider et al. (2010) described how staff often said their satisfaction in doing a good job enabled them to gain a sense of reward in what were often difficult circumstances. However, when staff began to find out more about a person's life, this altered their perception of that older person. We will be discussing how biographical information influences the staff approach to care in the following chapter.

Doing a good job

Write down your answers to the following questions:

- What brought you into working with older people?
- How would you define doing a 'good job'?
- What motivates you to do a good job?
- How would you define doing a good job when working with an older person?

Culture of safety

The culture of many organisations tends to be influenced by organisational philosophy and institutional constraints within the wider health and social care sector. The target-driven culture of the NHS means that acute NHS trusts tend to focus on the metrics of care (Patterson et al., 2011), which is not dissimilar to the long-term care industry, which is highly regulated with a predominately semi-skilled workforce (Anderson et al., 2003). Such organisations tend to favour a rule-based culture, where everyone is encouraged to think and act in a similar manner (Anderson et al., 2003).

In my research, leadership was a pivotal factor in the approaches to care adopted within each organisation (Brown Wilson, 2009). An individualised task-centred approach to care tended to be reinforced by a manager who could be described as 'leading from the front'. This has also been described as authoritarian in acute contexts where it was considered a good thing to keep staff trying their best (Patterson et al., 2011). 'Leading from the front' provided a clear structure where staff knew what was expected and they then structured individual routines around the risk management requirements for each resident. This focus meant that senior staff allocated work primarily by task so they could identify that the care had been given by the end of the shift. Teamwork in this case meant everyone pulling their weight, making sure the care was delivered. This is similar to how nurses in the acute sector manage the pace and complexity of their workload when required to meet targets such as discharging older patients from the ward before 10am (Patterson et al., 2011: 112).

Practice scenario: Care homes (Brown Wilson, 2007)

One manager described how recent involvement in a coroner's case had reinforced the importance of ensuring that appropriate risk assessments were undertaken; this meant she now advised all staff of changes through memos, so there was a clear record. The result of this was that staff were often directed to undertake specific tasks which rein-forced the individualised task-centred approach within the clinical environment. The (often) well-intentioned mantra of asking people to stay seated or directing them back to a position of safety prevents older people from engaging in meaningful activities, reinforcing dependence within that environment.

As we can see from the above case study, safety is often a well-intentioned aspect of care that tends to drive nursing towards a focus on the task. With a greater focus on effectiveness of health care services, there has also been an increasing focus on risk assessments (to ensure we are delivering appropriate care) combined with the focus on clinical outcomes (such as reducing falls), which has resulted in the development of a risk-averse culture in many environments caring for older people.

The (unrecognised) contribution of older people and their families

It remains clear that older people and their families in acute hospitals still have low expectations of care (Tadd et al., 2011). This was also evident in some of the units within my research where families felt that staff only had time to undertake the fundamental tasks of care. This low level of expectation was most evident when staff adopted an individualised task-centred approach. Families would offer to help with mealtimes for example, to make sure their relative received the care and support they needed. When staff focused on the practical nature of the caring tasks, these contributions were interpreted as helping them to 'get the job done'. Relationships with families were also influenced by the dominant focus on the tasks of caring, with many families describing how they made sure care was delivered.

ACTIVITY

Contributions of the older person and their family

- List how older people contribute to care in your care environment
- List the contributions families make in your care environment

Keep this list, as we will be building on this as we progress through the following chapters.

Older people contribute towards their care in ways often not recognised by staff who may be focused on the task, albeit in an individualised way; for example, an older person may begin to get undressed by undoing buttons, or removing jewellery to help staff save time. It was also during my research that I began to see how older people used personal stories to contribute to their care. Narratives and patient stories are beginning to be used as a mechanism for relaying the lived experience of a condition. Older people and their families share stories with staff who care for them across the different contexts of health and social care. This is often considered interesting but might not be included as part of the care planning process.

In seminars I have led, students recounted from practice anecdotes shared by older people that changed the student's perception of the person. Information shared by the older person often challenged the students' assumptions about the abilities or interests of older people. This enabled the student to see the older person as someone able to make their own decisions. But when asked how they use this information to shape care, the students stated it was not something they had considered. This was similar to the attitudes of staff who adopted an individualised task-centred approach in my research, who described the stories they heard from older people as interesting but did not see them as an active contribution being made by the older person or their family. For example, one care worker explained how he had learned that one of the women he cared for had been a school teacher and would turn off the lights each time she left the communal lounge room. This helped him to understand why she turned off the lights but it did not influence any other aspects of her care. This suggests that when we become focused on the task, we may filter out information that we don't think is relevant, such as biographical information or stories and anecdotes people may share about their life. In my research, sharing personal information seemed to be the key in supporting staff to move towards a person-centred approach. However, staff also needed to recognise the significance of this information before a person-centred approach could be enacted.

Summary

An individualised task-centred approach to care might occur when:

- New members of staff are getting to know the routines and how they need to do the task they have been assigned
- Staff are getting to know an older person when they first enter a service
- Members of staff believe this is the best way to deliver good-quality care to everyone in their care
- During staff shortages so that care can be delivered to a minimum standard
- When agency staff are employed, as individual preferences for an older person can be communicated quickly and easily, ensuring individualised care

Conclusion

We have seen from this chapter that older people often use care routines to provide information about themselves to staff by sharing personal stories. This may be a mechanism whereby the older person communicates to staff what is important to them in maintaining their 'self' in light of changing physical and cognitive abilities. Actively sharing stories with staff might suggest that older people prefer a more personal level of care. Families also demonstrate this by seeking out staff, showing their interest and discussing ways of supporting staff in the care of their relative. Listening to this information and understanding its significance to both the older person and the care being delivered will support us in moving to a person-centred approach to care. Staff who are able to recognise the significance of the biographical information being shared, and then act on this information, are more likely to adopt a person-centred approach.

CHAPTER 3

Focusing on the person

Learning outcomes

By the end of this the chapter, the reader will be able to:

- Describe how person-centred care might be implemented by more in-depth knowledge about an older person's life
- Develop practical strategies that would promote person-centred care in their practice
- Evaluate the differences between an individualised task-centred approach and a person-centred approach to care
- Critically examine how motivation to care might impact on how staff approach their care
- Consider how the contribution of older people and their supporters might influence the care process

Introduction

In Chapter 1, I outlined the conceptual development of the terms 'patient-centred' and 'person-centred' care, demonstrating that many of these terms had been developed in different contexts for different reasons. Person-centred care is becoming part of established policy, but a number of UK-based studies still demonstrate that achieving these concepts in practice remains an aspiration rather than a reality (Goodrich and Cornwell, 2008; Brooker et al., 2011; Patterson et al., 2011; Tadd et al., 2011). It may be that many of the person-centred care models are based on principles and it might not always be clear how these principles can be transferred into practice.

In the previous chapter, we considered how to provide good clinical care, individualised to the person. In this chapter, we are going to consider how a person-centred approach might improve the experience of older people. The approach outlined in this chapter is based on the 'resident-centred care' described in my research (Brown Wilson and Davies, 2009). For this chapter, I have reviewed the processes of 'resident-centred care' alongside the models of person-centred care outlined in Chapter 1 to ensure parity with the underlying principles of other models of person-centred care. In undertaking this review, it became evident that the processes described in my research provided the mechanism by which the principles of person-centred care might be enacted (Figure 3.1).

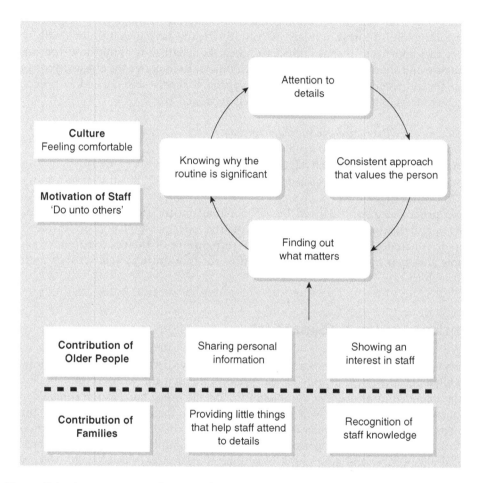

Figure 3.1 A person-centred approach to care

The person-centred approach presented in this chapter moves beyond considering the 'what' of care, such as a person's likes or dislikes, to the 'why' of care. Implementing what might appear as small details to a professional are integrally important to the quality of care and quality of life for an older person. Understanding why different details are significant in a person's life may also provide insights into how a person manages their health. For example, knowing how someone has approached their life as a younger person will provide insights into why they make the decisions they do as an older person. As we discussed in the previous chapter, this information may be provided informally by older people or their supporters in the stories they share with staff, but might not be recognised as important. There were times in my research where these details were missed from a person's routine because not all staff saw the significance of them.

Person-centred care, as outlined in this chapter, is about making it clear to all members of staff why information is important and how it might be integrated into decision making. I am sure many of you are already saying that, individually, you adopt this approach. If that is the case, then this chapter is about how you might formalise and share this good practice with others, to improve the consistency of the older person receiving a person-centred approach across shifts. The key processes which contribute towards a person-centred approach are:

- Finding out what matters to the older person
- Knowing why the routine is significant
- Attention to details based on this information
- Adopting a consistent approach that values the person

These processes are influenced by the personal motivation of staff to 'do unto others', and the dominant culture of making the older person feel comfortable. The chapter concludes by looking at how the recognition of the contribution of older people and their families might move staff towards adopting a relationship-centred approach to care.

Finding out what matters

When you read a biography of a person, it is generally written by another person who will highlight important aspects of that person's life that the writer thinks is relevant to the intended audience. An autobiography on the other hand is the person's own account of their life and as such will identify issues in their life that are important to them as an individual. A similar distinction might also be drawn between undertaking a life history with an older person, which is autobiographical and adopts a chrono-logical perspective, and adopting a biographical approach in assessment, which will focus on issues relevant to the professional undertaking the assessment. However, I do not believe that these approaches are mutually exclusive and we might adopt strategies relevant to both activities in order to develop a person-centred approach.

Assessment and care planning tend to be professionally driven, taking regulatory requirements into account. Nurses may undertake an assessment with an older person but then move off to devise a care plan relevant to their professional expectations of what this older person may or may not be able to achieve while in their care. This will often be derived from previous experience of older people and their own pre-conceived ideas as to what a person 'of this age' might hope to achieve. This may result in an individualised plan of care focusing on goals the professional feels 'ought to be achieved'. However, this may then result in an individualised task-centred approach as these goals are often defined in terms of caregiving tasks (personal hygiene, mobility, nutrition, etc.). These goals may not represent what is important from the perspective of the older person.

Amanda Clarke identified the importance of biographical information when considering the choices older people made as they aged (Clarke, 2000). A biographical approach emphasises that the attitudes, desires and interests of older people are a culmination of life experience, and views later decades as a time of ongoing development and self-determination. Adopting a biographical approach encourages older people to talk about their life experiences, enabling us to gain a fuller appreciation of people's needs, concerns and aspirations (Clarke et al., 2003). This is particularly important when we care for people with dementia, as identified in the following case study.

Practice scenario: Care homes (Brown Wilson, 2007)

Mary would always become anxious in the afternoon, at the time when children were being collected from school. She would search for a way out and become increasingly distressed. When staff would tell her that her children were now grown up, Mary would become suspicious as she did not believe the staff. One staff member, on seeing her distress, would spend a few minutes sitting with Mary and her photo album, showing her pictures of her children over the years to a recent holiday they had spent together. This relieved Mary's anxiety and helped her feel more comfortable in the home.

Belinda Dewar (2011) recounts a similar story in an acute ward where a woman with dementia who had worked in the beauty section of a department store was becoming agitated, looking for a way out, so staff asked if she would like to give them a hand massage, which relieved this person's anxiety. These two examples demonstrate how staff saw the situation from the perspective of the older person and used biographical knowledge to identify an action that created a positive social environment.

A biographical approach considers the aspirations of the older person and not simply what might be achieved in the immediate timeframe. Considering how a person approached their life prior to becoming older may provide additional insights into how older people maintain their sense of personal identity during the ageing process (Clarke and Warren, 2007). The following practice scenario demonstrates how undertaking a routine task such as changing a wound dressing can lead to older people sharing personal information about themselves. It also demonstrates why it is important that we recognise the relevance of this biographical information to the care of the older person and consider ways of creating a more personalised and responsive approach using this information. Considering the personal expectations of the older person within the assessment process may challenge how we view our professional role.

Practice scenario: Community

Mary came to have her wound dressed in a clinic. While the staff nurse was getting the appropriate wound dressing, the student began speaking with Mary. The student found out Mary had sustained the wound from a fall in her garden. She had been very active previously and was beginning to feel quite down as she no longer felt safe in leaving her home or working in her garden due to her fear of falling. Although from the professional perspective, wound management was the key problem, the student realised that for Mary herself, the main problem was her fear of falling. This information was used to refer Mary to the community falls team, where she was able to attend classes to regain her confidence and reduce the likelihood of future falls.

A starting point in implementing a person-centred approach might be to use a common nursing framework such as the activities of living developed by Roper, Logan and Tierney (2001), and consider how questions might be framed to provide the older person with the opportunity to share information about themselves. This may support an older person in communicating information they might not have thought would be of interest to the professional. For example, when asking about mobility we might consider asking where an older person walks, whether they exercise for necessity or pleasure, where they do their shopping and how they travel there. By asking these questions we might discover that an older person lives some distance from shopping facilities and so needs to continue to be able to drive a car. In her study in acute sector wards, Belinda Dewar (2011) implemented a questionnaire that supported staff in finding out what matters to the individual; patients and relatives were quite surprised to be included in discussions in this way but patients expressed they would not 'feel silly' about saying something that was on their mind later in their stay. We will look at this in more detail in Chapter 6.

As the baby boomer generation ages, we are seeing a change in how older people are living out their later years. This will also change their aspirations and expectations of what they wish to achieve as they age. As nurses we need to consider what might be important to older people such as issues surrounding their sexuality and how this is expressed; how older people view their own spirituality and how this might differ from the practice of religion. Older people are being encouraged to maintain more active and varied lifestyles, which will have an impact on what constitutes meaningful activity, as we see more people becoming involved in walking clubs, gyms, and dance and exercise classes. The challenge for professionals is to consider how this information might be accessed and used within the health and social care encounter.

Knowing the person

Draw a table with three columns:

- In the first column, list the biographical information shared by an older person during personal care routines
- In the second column, list how information might be relevant to this person's care routines
- In the third column, list what further action this information might require of you

Now compare this table with the table you prepared in the Chapter 2 activity: Developing an individualised plan of care. What are the key differences for the older person's care routine and why do you think these differences might be significant to the older person?

Knowing why the routine is significant

As we discussed in Chapter 2, we all have a routine to our daily life. This routine is influenced by life events, the job we might have done, family life and where we have lived. While our routines may change, we often keep that which is familiar to us and gives our life meaning. Zisberg et al. (2007) suggest that personal routines reflect not only a person's lifestyle but also their identity, and that maintaining personal routines at a time of major life change is an important challenge for nursing that could have positive benefits for people requiring care. Cook and Brown Wilson (2010) recount how older people can be supported in maintaining activities that give their life meaning, such as picking blackberries in the summer months. The following practice scenario demonstrates how staff on busy wards can also support older people in undertaking meaningful routines and so make a valued contribution to the care environment.

Practice scenario: Medical unit

One woman missed having bacon rolls and being able to read the newspaper, so staff went to the canteen each day to get her a bacon roll and made sure she had access to her usual newspaper. In return, this woman wanted to help, so staff found jobs that helped them, such as folding bags. The woman enjoyed doing this. (Dewar, 2011)

From a professional perspective, such routines might not be of great significance, particularly in acute care, but continuing meaningful activity promotes the older person's wellbeing and quality of life. This suggests that knowing how a person undertakes their personal routine at home is a first step in understanding why it is significant to that person.

Understanding why a routine is significant enables professionals to prioritise their care, taking the knowledge of this routine into account. Communicating this information to all members of the nursing team will ensure a consistent approach. For example, knowing when an older person is likely to get up in the night to access the toilet is a vital piece of information when they are in an unfamiliar environment. If an older person is unable to get out of bed and find their way easily, this might cause anxiety, agitation and distress from subsequent incontinence. This is particularly important for people with dementia who might not be able to communicate what they usually do, but become quite agitated or upset when they are unable to continue important routines.

Routines are not only about personal care but may also include meaningful activity older people engaged in across their day – for instance, instrumental activities of daily living (such as housework, cooking, gardening, etc.) or enjoyable pastimes (such as attending dances, swimming, being involved in activities with the family and wider community). A student recounted one story where an older woman shared her love of salsa dancing and how she hoped to be able to get back to it. This insight prompted the student to get in touch with the physiotherapist so that her therapy could take this into account.

Deteriorating health should not be a reason not to engage in meaningful activity or pleasurable past times. Understanding what a person used to do will provide professionals with insights into the support older people might need to continue to undertake activities that give their lives meaning. For example, a survey of home care services found that person-centred care was often about facilitating activities that enabled older people to leave their home as this was an aspect of life that they valued (Patmore and McNulty, 2005).

Attention to detail

We all feel good about ourselves when we know we look our best and it is no different for an older person, irrespective of the health care environment they find themselves in. Considering important details from the perspective of the older person and facilitating their inclusion into the care regime is fundamental to adopting a person-centred approach. Attention to detail might be as simple as ensuring the person is dressed in clothing the family have brought in, supporting an older man to shave or an older woman to apply makeup and put on their jewellery. Such attention to detail, as recounted in the following practice scenario, should be seen as part of the routine and not as something extra we are asking of staff. Capturing this information is not always easy in records but it is essential if we are to adopt a person-centred approach consistently and so provide care that matters to each person.

> ## Practice scenario: Care home (Brown Wilson, 2007)
>
> Freda told me how important it was that she could tell the time. Following her stroke, she was unable to see the clock on the wall so it was important to have her watch on each day. Staff understood this was important because Freda had been a teacher who was always prepared in advance of things happening. Knowing when something was about to happen, such as when the tea trolley was due, remained an important feature of her life. Staff had listened to these stories and identified how this information might be applied into Freda's everyday care routines. This biographical detail seemed to be an integral part of implementing person-centred care.

Older people and their families often share anecdotes or stories about their lives, which might not always appear relevant in a busy health care environment. This volunteering of personal information is an important contribution, as it enables staff to build up a store of personal information that might be used to understand why a person might be behaving in a certain way. Men who have been prisoners of war, for example, might find being in dark and confined spaces difficult and react in ways that are uncharacteristic for them. Someone who has worked on a farm all their life and is used to being up before dawn to milk cows might still be getting up at this hour and require a cup of tea, for example, rather than being told they need to return to bed. Having access to biographical information supports professionals in being responsive to the older person's needs. Tadd et al. (2011) recount how one member of staff engaged with a woman about her interests in gardening during her meal, which meant that this lady enjoyed her meal. In my research, I observed care staff similarly engaging older people with stories during assistance with meals. There was one older woman who regularly refused her meals but when staff engaged in social conversation during the meal about what she had cooked for her family and the food she enjoyed in her life, mealtimes became a pleasurable occasion for everyone involved. Biographical details support us in looking beyond immediate needs, identifying what might be behind the behaviour rather than making a judgement based solely on the immediate behaviour.

Professionals who only see the immediate needs might be operating within the remit of a time-limited service that is increasingly coming under financial pressure. Being aware of the assumptions we make is the first step in ensuring that an older person's needs are being placed at the centre of the process and that our professional decisions are not precluding older people from opportunities to return to a good quality of life that incorporates meaningful activities. This is support that meets the person's needs in ways that matter to them.

A consistent approach that values the person

Understanding how someone has lived their life previously will enable professionals to see beyond immediate needs and incorporate an older person's goals or aspirations into health care decisions. Involving older people in decisions can at times be challenging as eyesight and hearing might deteriorate over time. Older people may also take longer in processing information but while this does not mean they can't understand, it does mean we need to give them more time to assimilate the information. This may be why many older people ask friends or family to come with them when meeting with professionals, because they feel they might not hear or be able to follow what is being said due to the speed at which the encounter is conducted, as demonstrated in the following practice scenario.

Practice scenario: Medical unit

Mr Smith was considered to be grumpy and bad-tempered following transfer to the unit. The student began speaking to Mr Smith and found he was pleasant and easy to talk to. In their discussions, Mr Smith told the student that in being moved between wards, he had lost his hearing aid and now struggled to hear what was being said to him, which he said made him bad-tempered. The student communicated this to the ward team who were then able to change their communication with Mr Smith to involve him in decisions being made in his care.

Many (but not all) older people experience presbycusis (or age-related hearing loss). This syndrome includes:

- Reduced hearing acuity
- High frequency hearing loss
- Difficulties understanding speech in noise
- Slowed processing of acoustic information
- Impaired localisation of sound source (Tolson et al., 2011: 140)

The emotional impact that not being able to hear might have on older people is often not recognised and could be resolved by effective communication strategies (Tolson and Brown Wilson, 2011). When in the community, many older people may require consultation and/or clinical appointments. It is important that when older people require hearing aids they are supported to use them effectively. Many consulting rooms now have a loop system that facilitates this. If written material is part of the consultation process, knowing people require glasses and ensuring these are cleaned and well fitting is another aspect of facilitating involvement. Although hearing aids can improve the disabling effects of hearing loss, they do not completely reduce this disability. This means that health care professionals need to give the older person time to assimilate information, which might include giving it in smaller segments so there is time to absorb the information.

This strategy needs to be recognised by professionals who might need to consider how they communicate with older people. Having supporters with them gives older people the security that there is someone who is promoting their best interests, but such supporters should not be used as a proxy when older people are still able to make their own decisions. Assuming older people will not understand the decisions required of them is the most common form of perpetuation of ageism across health and social care. A biographical approach to assessment and care planning is the first step in breaking down these assumptions and the barriers they cause for older people's involvement in decision making about issues that impact on their lives.

We can see the importance of biographical details in developing a person-centred approach to care but capturing biographical details in nursing records in a way that is meaningful remains a challenge. A life history document might be useful for staff, but this does not replace key information which could influence a person's care becoming part of their care plan. Different strategies will need to be adopted in different areas of practice. These need to be flexible yet relevant to the communication required in the health or social care environment, as biographical information ensures we include the voice of older people in the planning of their care. The role of the nurse is pivotal to ensure this information is shared with other professionals within the multi-disciplinary team. Nurses can identify the relevant details and how these will positively impact on the care of the older person and then present this in a way that the rest of the team can appreciate and assimilate into the decision-making process.

Understanding an older person's biography will also enable nurses to consider how we might support older people to participate in decisions that affect them. For example, an older woman who has lived on her own for some time might be very used to making her own decisions and may resent others doing this on her behalf. Assuming older people do not want to or are unable to participate in the decision-making process undermines their sense of who they are and subsequently their dignity. On the other hand, finding ways of supporting the participation of older people in decisions that matter to them demonstrates we are treating them with dignity as we promote their ability to make their own decisions (autonomy) (Bayer et al., 2005).

The culture of making a person 'comfortable'

In my research, for person-centred care to develop, staff described how they might approach care as you would in a person's own home. While there was the recognition from staff that a care home has become the person's own home, many older people did not see it as their home. However, staff also described how it was important for people to feel as comfortable as they would in their own home. Sharing personal information was important in developing personal and responsive relationships that helped everyone feel comfortable within the environment. This was also reflected in Belinda Dewar's (2011) work in the acute sector, where sharing personal information helped develop personal relationships with patients and relatives. In the community, one woman would make her own lunch so there was time for the care worker to take her out of the house, because this is what was important to her (Patmore and McNulty, 2005).

Staff who describe adopting a person-centred approach also describe a 'do unto others' philosophy in their care, where their motivation was to 'make a difference' when providing care. In my research, doing unto others means doing what the older person wants, because that is what staff would like for themselves. This is a different perspective from that expressed in other studies. For example, other care homes research highlights 'the golden rule' in terms of how care is delivered to 'me' or 'my family' (Anderson et al., 2005). A similar motivation was also described in Belinda Dewar's (2011) study where staff made assumptions about the way people wanted care to be delivered.

Adopting a person-centred approach moves beyond doing 'a good job' in terms of clinical care to considering the implications of receiving care from the older person's perspective. In care homes, Flesner and Rantz (2004) suggest that giving direct care staff the authority to make decisions about how to spend their time enables them to support residents in meeting life preferences and goals. Similarly, others have shown that in home care, staff who knew the aspirations of the person they cared for and became motivated to fulfil these aspirations were able to provide person-centred care in ways that often required little extra time (Patmore and McNulty, 2005). Staff who described this motivation also talked about how they contributed to making a person feel comfortable.

Contributions of older people and families

The stories older people share might not be valued by them or their families when presented with the professional perspective. However, it is not possible to undertake a biographical approach without this knowledge. By valuing this knowledge, we are also communicating that we value the older person and their supporters. Understanding and acting on these significant details shows we respect what is important to the older person, which is a key tenet of promoting a person's dignity. When considering a biographical approach, hearing the voice of the older person and their families will ensure we are implementing a person-centred approach. While it is important to recognise the value of information shared with us, families also work very hard to support the older person in undertaking meaningful activities. This contribution may go unrecognised by staff as it is not as visible as practical care.

Summary

A person-centred approach to care might occur when staff:

- Respect the person and value their sense of identity
- Understand the significance of the biography to that person in their current place

- Transfer 'personal' knowledge to specific actions in care routines
- Understand the behaviour of the older person in the context of their changing abilities/ needs

Conclusion

As professionals we rarely have the luxury of considering only one person at a time. We are often confronted by competing priorities when caring for a group of people. This might be in a residential environment where we have a number of older people with a range of complex conditions requiring care simultaneously, or in caring for multiple people in their own home environments. A person-centred approach is something we are able to give on a one-to-one basis and is vital when we are in the care encounter. The next chapter describes another approach, which moves from a one-to-one focus to one that considers the issues for a *group* of older people, ensuring everyone receives a person-centred approach in spite of competing priorities. It is the recognition of the contribution being made by older people and their families that enables staff to move towards a relationship-centred approach.

CHAPTER 4

Focusing on relationships

Learning outcomes

By the end of this the chapter, the reader will be able to:

- Describe how the organisational context influences the care of older people
- Evaluate the difference between person-centred and relationship-centred approaches
- Develop practical strategies that enable the needs of older people, their supporters and staff to be considered in the decision-making process
- Critically examine the importance of leadership and teamwork in promoting a relationship-centred approach to care

Introduction

In Chapter 3, we considered how biographical knowledge enabled us to focus care on the person. This meant we considered details in care routines that held significance from the older person's perspective. It was also apparent in Chapter 3 how older people and their families contributed towards developing personal and responsive relationships with staff. This was different from the models we reviewed in Chapter 1, where the contribution of older people was implicit rather than explicit. However, there were times in my research where there were competing needs and priorities within the care environment, requiring a different approach to care. This approach was underpinned by shared understandings that contributed to decision making and reflected the perspectives of older people, families and staff. The importance of relationships between the older person, their families and staff is also a feature of person-centred care, but the needs of the older person remain central to the process and outcome of care. Relationship-centred care, however, considers the needs of everyone involved in the caring relationship (Figure 4.1).

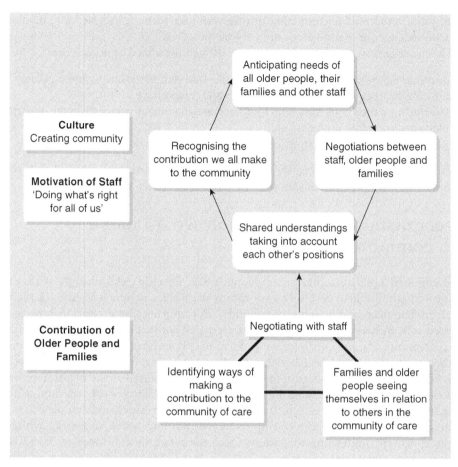

Figure 4.1   The relationship-centred approach

Relationship-centred care, as outlined in this chapter, is based on my research in long-term care (Brown Wilson and Davies, 2009), and considers how a person-centred approach might be achieved in communal care environments. For example, Belinda Dewar (2011) describes person-centred processes that contribute towards the development of compassionate relationship-centred care in hospital wards. In the preceding chapters, we saw how adopting an individualised task-centred approach might be described as the 'what' of care while adopting a person-centred approach explains the 'why'. Adopting a relationship-centred approach for the individual older person supports us in moving towards a more participatory way of working where the personhood of everyone in the relationship is considered (Nolan et al., 2004). A relationship-centred approach helps us understand the 'how' of care as it takes the organisational context into account, which also includes the needs of other older people, families and staff. The relationship-centred approach presented in this chapter recognises organisational constraints by highlighting the importance of negotiation to enable competing priorities of care to be recognised and managed to acknowledge the perspectives of everyone involved.

The processes involved in adopting a relationship-centred approach are:

- Anticipating the needs of older people, families and staff in the environment of care
- Creating strategies that include negotiation and compromise
- Developing shared understandings by acknowledging that all perspectives are important in the decision-making process
- Recognising the contribution each party makes to the community of care

These processes are influenced by leadership and teamwork that create a culture of community where the organisation of care takes all needs into account.

Recognising the contribution we all make to the community of care

In communal environments, older people often develop relationships with each other, and families also develop relationships with older people who are not related to them but part of the same community. Recognising these relationships is an important feature of understanding the diversity of contributions being made within the community of care. One relative spoke to me about how one of the other women in the care home would visit his grandmother, who preferred to stay in her room. This contribution meant his grandmother was not as isolated as she might have been and this was much appreciated by the family. Other relatives told me about how bringing their grandchildren into the home gave other residents added pleasure.

Developing reciprocal relationships and maintaining social networks while in hospital remain important to patients and their families. Bridges et al. (2010) referred to this as 'connect with me' and Dewar (2011) described how staff make connections through the use of humour and banter. Humour may be used on a number of levels, for example staff in care homes identify the importance of humour in developing reciprocal relationships with residents (Brown Wilson et al., 2009b) or it may be seen as a mechanism to relieve stress (Schneider et al., 2010). Certainly in my research, being involved in initiating or responding to humour helped families feel part of the wider community. For this to occur, staff recognised and valued the contribution made by both residents and families in humorous situations.

Practice scenario: Care home (Brown Wilson, 2007)

One care worker was particularly skilled at creating a sense of community and engagement as he went about his work. There were days when his approach resembled street theatre as he 'made an entrance' and then spoke to different residents as he passed

(Continued)

(Continued)

by, involving them in the conversation he was having with his colleagues in the room. This engaged the residents and their eyes lit up as they followed the movement and conversation as this member of staff moved around the room. Once he had left the room, many of the residents appeared more animated and were speaking to their neighbours.

Older people themselves may contribute to the community of care by helping other older people in the environment: one woman I spoke with told me how she would look out for a man who was newly admitted and let staff know when he needed help. This was not dissimilar to the contribution of a patient in Belinda Dewar's study who felt that staff appreciated her looking out for another patient in her bay (Dewar, 2011).

Practice scenario: Care home (Brown Wilson, 2007)

Freda told me how she always helped Gwen, who had poor hearing and poor sight. Gwen couldn't see what was happening across the room and so Freda would tell her who was in the room and convey the conversations to her so she could be involved. Gwen also struggled to hear what was on the menu and again Freda would tell her this. Freda felt she was helping her friend to remain in touch with what was happening in the home each day.

Staff recognising the contributions highlighted in the previous practice scenario are then able to facilitate relationships, contributing towards a culture of community (Brown Wilson, 2009).

Anticipating the needs of older people, families and staff

The flexibility and organisation of care was an important feature in the care environment where I observed a relationship-centred approach being enacted. In my research, I observed care being delivered in a person-centred way but this was only made possible by the organisation of care that took the needs of the older people, families and staff into account. Anticipation involved knowing the significant details for each of the residents and ensuring these were attended to, given the wider context of the workload. Anticipating needs helps with the planning of care, for example, in my research, staff told me how they knew when people liked to go to bed and when to get up, and subsequently planned the care to take these choices into account.

Practice scenario: Medical unit

Mr Raine required extensive bandaging to his legs, which was time-consuming and left the student worrying about the other patients she needed to attend to. It became evident that this patient really appreciated the opportunity to talk so the student reprioritised her work to leave this task until last, which ensured time to find out more about Mr Raine's interests and life story. They discovered mutual interests and Mr Raine's self-esteem was boosted by an appreciative audience.

Dewar (2011) also identifies how a member of staff prioritised their time on a busy shift to sit with an older woman with dementia so she was supported to drink sufficient fluids following treatment. Understanding that some older people may require more time when providing care is something that can be anticipated and factored into the general organisation of the ward (Patterson et al., 2011). Rather than make decisions in isolation, staff were seen to become involved in negotiation and compromise with each other, as well as involving older people and, where relevant, their families.

ACTIVITY

Return to the activity you completed in Chapter 1: Identifying the key priorities, where you prioritised 'other' tasks over the care of an older person and consider the following:

- Were the needs of the older person able to be anticipated?
- If so, how might you reorganise care to ensure the 'other' task and the needs of the older person were met?
- In future, how might you negotiate a compromise to ensure the needs of the older person, the family (where relevant) and staff are met?

Negotiation and compromise

When I observed staff negotiating with each other, they often referred to significant details that had alerted them to a developing problem with a resident, and then identified how they felt they had the right skills to deal with it before it caused distress. For example, staff did not sit back and allow others to persevere with a situation when it was becoming apparent that difficulties were arising, such as in the following practice scenario.

Practice scenario: Care home (Brown Wilson, 2007)

Bettina was refusing her lunch. A staff member whom I had observed successfully support Bettina at a previous mealtime was advising her colleague as to how best to approach the situation. As it became apparent that Bettina was becoming more distressed, the staff member suggested they swap positions, which was agreed. The staff member who had suggested they swap positions told me that some people were better at doing things than others and she knew she could get Bettina to eat her meal, so it made sense to do this and they both enjoyed the experience.

Staff who worked in this way described how they 'weighed up' the needs of each resident, the needs of the staff and the needs of the family according to the situation. I also observed staff discussing different compromises within the care routines with each other, so they could then discuss the options with the older people whose routines might be disrupted. For example, when one resident was unable to have a bath due to staff shortages one morning, her key worker realised the personal significance of this to the resident and negotiated changes in the schedule for the following morning. These residents and their families accepted the changed routines because they understood what was happening in the wider context of the home.

There were times, however, when families also needed to be involved in these negotiations. For example, one family member unexpectedly came to take her father out after lunch and had to wait for staff to change his clothing, which had become soiled during the meal. Staff explained how they had prioritised the care of other more frail residents at this time. The family member, accepting this explanation, agreed to ring to enable staff to alter their work planning for future occasions. Staff also agreed to consider how they might support this resident differently at mealtimes so he might not need changing on similar occasions. This is an example of working together to shape the way things are done. Such planning might at times require nurses to be led by the older person's perspective or that of the family, even though it might not be what you might consider, as a professional, to be the 'best way' of doing something (Dewar, 2011).

There may also be times when negotiation about roles is required to support older people in retaining or developing self-care. The following example suggests that for staff in acute care environments, negotiation and compromise mean spotting opportunities to work differently (Dewar, 2011).

Practice scenario: Medical unit (Dewar, 2011)

Some older people come into hospital and expect staff to do everything for them and don't realise they need to stay independent. Staff on one unit describe how they negotiated what needed to be done with one patient and how they sat and spoke with her to 'strike a deal' to encourage her independence.

Working in this way develops shared understandings between older people, families and staff. In my research, such understandings were often developed through narration of accounts, which can act as a powerful tool in communicating the values within a care environment (Ronch, 2004).

Shared understandings

Shared understandings emerge within the caring relationship as the contributions made by residents, families and staff are valued within the care environment. This may consist of personal stories, as discussed in Chapter 3, or it may include the ways of assisting discussed earlier in this chapter. These contributions lead to reciprocal relationships which are further developed by the negotiation and compromise that emerge within most care-giving environments. It is the shared understanding of the situation from the perspective of the older person, the families and staff that support shared decision making.

Patterson et al. (2011) suggest that shared understandings can be as simple as making time to talk to the older person and their family to make sure everyone has the same information, or it might involve meeting the needs of the families, such as providing them with a meal when they are visiting and making sure they have the support they need at home. In my research, staff members shared examples of everyday interactions with families, revealing how they understood the changing perspective of each family member, accommodating this perspective into the decisions being made. This is similar to carers in the community who may need to accommodate the needs of the family members as well as the needs of the person they care for (Clissett, 2007).

Practice scenario: Care homes (Brown Wilson, 2007)

Fiona was one family member who would visit the home each day to help care for her husband. She took great pride in making sure the staff had access to enough clothing for her husband. She understood the difficulties the staff faced and was rarely seen to be upset. One evening she came up to a member of staff very anxious and distressed because one of her husband's slippers had gone missing – these were new and had only just been bought. Although the staff member was busy, she recognised how important this was to Fiona and stopped what she was doing to locate the missing slipper, which they did. The staff member told me this was important because she recognised the contribution made by Fiona with her husband's clothing.

A relationship-centred approach supports reciprocal relationships where older people and families are seen as active contributors to the community of care (Brown Wilson et al., 2009b). When older people and families are involved in the decision-making process, staff may also expect shared understandings. For example, a senior care worker in my research was disappointed when it became apparent that an older woman had spoken to another caregiver about the care on one of his shifts where they had been very busy. This senior care worker felt that as staff had involved the resident in the decision-making process, this woman might have been more understanding. In this way there was an expectation that this older woman would take into account the perspective of staff. I also observed examples where other residents recognised the communal routine and acknowledged that staff needed to attend to others before them. There were also times when older people and families would alter their expectations of care by taking into account the perspectives of staff. This was not to say they accepted poor care but that they recognised when changes had to be made to the usual routines. Tadd et al. (2011) also recount stories where older people and families saw the pressure staff were working under in acute services and subsequently accepted care being delivered differently. In my study, older people and families often accepted changes to their routines as they knew when staff were able, they would return to the usual pattern of care delivery that ensured significant details were attended to. Families who made a contribution that was intended to benefit those in the wider community of care, demonstrated an understanding of the needs of others within the care environment. This contributed towards a shared understanding of how staff worked, which meant they accepted staff decisions about care priorities. One family member told me that he knew that when his father needed help, staff would not walk past him, and so he was prepared to accept when other residents might need more help than his father on certain days. In acute environments, information sharing is an important feature of developing shared understandings and Dewar (2011) suggests that the use of language helps people to feel connected. One family member, for example, remarked how a consultant asking her opinion on how her mother was, made her feel her contribution was valued. This suggests that as shared understandings develop, the recognition of everyone's contribution to the community of care is enhanced, which in itself perpetuates the cycle of relationship-centred care.

A culture of community

Care environments may not always lend themselves to the idea of being a community. I have argued previously (Brown Wilson, 2009) that it might be of greater value to consider care homes as communities rather than as a person's own home. That is not to say that we should not try to make older people feel 'at home' in these environments, but that we should recognise the breadth of relationships that exist within communal care environments. I would also suggest that acute wards would benefit from being considered as communities of care. For example, in their systematic literature review and meta synthesis, Bridges et al. identify the importance of feeling connected to others when on acute wards and considered that 'creating community' was a theme of importance to older people and their families across studies in acute hospitals:

> The review's findings highlight how an acute care episode necessitates the creation of new connections and that these, plus the maintenance of existing connections, provide the community through which enriched care can be delivered. (2010: 105)

For reciprocal relationships to develop, staff need to be able to see all perspectives in the relationship. 'Doing what's right for all of us' sometimes meant focusing on the need of the older person, but there were also times when it meant focusing on the need of the family members, as highlighted by the following practice scenario.

Practice scenario: Care home (Brown Wilson, 2007)

Each time Elisabeth visited her husband, she had a routine where, at the end of her visit, she would come up to each member of staff and thank them for looking after her husband. She would then walk to the door of the locked unit to say her goodbyes. There was another resident who would always try to use this as an opportunity to leave the unit, which would disrupt Elisabeth's chance to say farewell to her husband. The staff understood the importance of this and so would distract the other woman to enable Elisabeth to have this private time with her husband uninterrupted. This meant the visit ended in a way that enabled Elisabeth to feel comfortable once she had left her husband. Families experiencing this approach often acknowledged their appreciation to the staff involved.

When staff regularly adopted a relationship-centred approach, they appreciated when older people and families acknowledged their perspective but did not expect this from everyone. One care worker, for example, spoke about her personal philosophy as wanting to give something back as she didn't know if she may need similar care in the future. For staff working in the acute sector, adopting a relationship-centred approach often requires them to deviate from the usual pattern of working. Dewar (2011) suggests that staff need to be courageous and open to the opportunities of doing things differently but also need to connect to their own feelings about the situation. I observed staff who consistently adopted a relationship-centred approach, exchanging information informally with each other, which enabled them to speak about their feelings and feel supported by their team members. Staff in the community often work alone, with feelings of connection arising from a familiarity with the client and family member (Clissett, 2007).

It was evident in my research that it was possible for some staff to recognise and respond to the perspective of older people and families in isolated instances. However, for this approach to be consistently adopted within one caring environment, such as a care home, a critical mass of staff who adopt the same approach is required. From my observations of staff, it was evident that the critical mass of staff shared a similar motivation for being in care work, such as 'doing a good job' for an individualised, task-centred approach and 'making a difference' in a person-centred approach. This may account for why in acute trusts, there can be very positive leadership within the organisation at a strategic level, but then impoverished wards exist at the local level. Conversely, there may be poor leadership within the wider organisation but very good practice on local units (Patterson et al., 2011). In my research, staff working together who shared the motivation of 'making a difference' certainly adopted person-centred practices and were more likely to consider working in more flexible ways that enabled a relationship-centred approach. For a relationship-centred approach to work consistently, the style and level of leadership was crucial (Brown Wilson, 2009).

The importance of leadership within health and social care environments cannot be overestimated and there are many texts that consider leadership styles and it is outside the scope of this book to critique these. My main concern when considering some of the leadership literature was the confusion between the terms 'leadership' and 'management'. While these are certainly overlapping concepts and it is important for managers to show leadership, other staff can also be leaders in health and social care environments. For a relationship-centred approach to be enacted, there needs to be a visible role modelling of person-centred approaches. For example, one newly employed care worker told me that when he was unsure of how to approach a resident, he would ask the senior care worker who then role modelled the best way of working with that person. This supported the staff member to get to know the significant details for each person and why they were important in daily routines. In her model of compassionate relationship-centred care, Belinda Dewar (2011) outlines the development of personal knowledge with the associated person-centred processes of 'knowing who I am and what matters to me' as crucial in relationship-centred care. Dewar (2011) suggests compassionate conversations as the mechanism by which this process moves towards working together to shape how care is delivered. While this provides individual staff with a mechanism to achieve a relationship-centred approach, there also needs to be support from the wider team (Patterson et al., 2011).

My research suggests that there need to be complementary tiers of leadership. This starts with a visible management tier, that is, role modelling good practice and creating an ethos of teamwork. Relationship-oriented leadership (Anderson et al., 2003) has been described as fostering interconnections and enhancing the information flow needed for flexible working practices (Table 4.1). I observed this style of leadership in my research, where staff were encouraged to share anecdotes about how different residents were throughout the morning with the nurse in charge. This meant that as the day progressed, everyone was able to alter their workload to take into account the changing needs of the residents.

Table 4.1 Attributes of a relationship-oriented leader (adapted from Anderson et al., 2003)

Being approachable
Generating trust
Giving constructive feedback
Helping staff resolve conflict
Promoting an exchange of information in decision making
Enabling staff to say what they mean without fear of retribution

While a central leader is important, my research suggests that for the flexible working patterns required by negotiation and compromise, care staff also need to be 'leading by example'. This is particularly important at a time when nursing responsibilities seem to be taking nurses further away from the bedside. When I observed leadership from care workers adopting a relationship-centred approach, there was informal communication between all workers that captured important details for the older person during that shift that enabled all levels of workers to adjust their care, involving older people and families in opportunities for negotiation. I believe a key nursing responsibility is to engage care workers in considering the perspectives of older people and families and then supporting these care workers in developing leadership skills to promote a relationship-centred approach to care. This is the first step to ensuring a culture of community where all perspectives are shared and valued.

Summary

A relationship-centred approach includes:

- Anticipation of individual residents' needs in the context of the needs of other residents and organisational demands or constraints
- Valuing the contribution of other staff, residents and families
- Negotiation – valuing all perspectives and being prepared to compromise
- Developing knowledge of how we all contribute towards the communal environment, leading to shared understandings with others

Conclusion

Relationships are integral to the care encounter, as we have seen in the preceding chapters. Each approach facilitates different types of relationships. Relationship-centred care with its focus on negotiation and shared decision making promotes reciprocal relationships. Reciprocity is about giving something back and an older person might be engaged in giving something back to staff such as a smile, a thank you or helping out with their care. This is the contribution we recognise from older people and their supporters in person-centred approaches. Reciprocal relationships in the context of relationship-centred care, as described in this chapter, means staff are facilitating opportunities for reciprocal engagement with older people, families and staff themselves, valuing the perspectives and needs of everyone in the relationship. It is this that enables staff to engage in strategies which promote a relationship-centred approach to care.

CHAPTER 5

Consequences of care: integrating the perspective of older people and families into the quality debate

Learning outcomes

By the end of this the chapter, the reader will be able to:

- Describe the consequences for the older person when different approaches to care are adopted
- Critically examine the mechanisms that potentially impact on the consequences for older people in different care environments
- Evaluate how these mechanisms might be altered to improve the consequences for older people, families and staff in different care environments
- Develop practical strategies that may improve the user experience by increasing the participation of older people, their families and supporters in the decision-making process

Introduction

In Chapter 1 we considered that there were different models of care that encouraged participation in different ways and that there might not be a 'one size fits all' model.

We then considered the process behind three broad approaches: an individualised task-centred, a person-centred and a relationship-centred approach. Each of these approaches requires a different focus of care and is influenced not only by the motivation of staff to adopt these approaches but also by structural factors such as leadership, continuity of staff and the culture of the caring environment. The discussion within each chapter inferred that there were consequences of adopting the different approaches, but these were not explicitly discussed. This chapter considers how the consequence for older people, families and staff might be considered when adopting different approaches to care and discusses how we might use this information to improve the experience of older people, families and staff in care environments.

While my research suggests that care homes might adopt an overall approach to care, there were also times when constraints within the care environment meant that staff might have to alter their practice. For me, this was most noticeable in the environment that adopted a primarily relationship-centred approach; for example, there were times when agency staff were required and so staff were not able to work as flexibly or involve older people, families or staff in the usual pattern of negotiation and compromise. This meant that established staff moved to a primarily individualised task-centred approach to ensure the clinical care was delivered. Residents, families and staff who experienced and delivered a primarily relationship-centred approach, felt the individualised task-centred approach was the bottom line of care, enabling them to deliver good-quality care but not always attending to significant details.

Alternatively, in environments where an individualised task-centred approach was dominant, staff spoke about the rewards of doing a good job with residents and families, expressing satisfaction at the care being delivered. When staff then attended to small details that went beyond clinical care to take into account things that made a difference to the experience of their day, families described this as unexpected when they acknowledged the heavy workload experienced by staff. However, in these environments, I observed one team delivering a person-centred and occasionally a relationship-centred approach, when working under the same organisational constraints.

Where I observed a primarily person-centred approach, attention to detail was described by staff as important because it made a difference to the experience of the older person. Families also spoke about how these details mattered and appreciated staff accommodating them into everyday routines. I observed that it was possible for staff members to deliver this approach in isolation to other team members. This was not possible with a relationship-centred approach, as the team needed to work together in a way that enabled them to adapt their care more flexibly when required. Also, the language used by caregivers to describe a relationship-centred approach differed in that it reflected engagement between staff, older people and families. This often went beyond information giving to demonstrate involvement in the decisions being made.

These insights prompted me to undertake further analysis of the data from my research. I reviewed interview transcripts from older people, families and staff for statements inferring judgements about both clinical care and the processes identified in the preceding three chapters. These judgements described the consequences for the older person, families and staff. Although consequences had emerged as an original theme, the further analysis extended these original themes to consider how they might represent a statement that described the experience of the older person when staff adopted a particular approach to care. From this analysis, three statements emerged that described how the consequences of each of the different approaches to care were experienced by older people (Table 5.1).

Table 5.1 The experience of care from the perspective of older people, families and staff

Theme: Approach to care	Theme: Consequences	Theme: Experience of care
Individualised task-centred	The most you can expect versus the bottom line	Care that satisfies me
Person-centred	Feeling cared for because details matter	Care that matters to me
Relationship-centred	Developing shared understandings by being involved in negotiation and compromise	Care that involves us all

Table 5.1 suggests that the approach being driven by the task is less positive to the experience of older people and families when compared to a more participatory approach. I suggested in Chapter 1 that the focus on the task, the person and the relationship provided differing opportunities for participation for the older person, families and staff and that one single model might not meet the needs of all stakeholders. This means that staff might adopt different approaches at different times depending on the people involved and the context of care. Using the judgements made by older people, families and staff in my research, I initially developed a hierarchy based on the experience of older people, families and staff (Brown Wilson, 2011). A hierarchy infers that you build from the bottom up, but it doesn't necessarily provide a mechanism to move down again. The idea of different approaches infers that care could move between approaches. Therefore, it might be more appropriate to consider the approaches in a step model (Figure 5.1), where we can move between the different approaches to care,

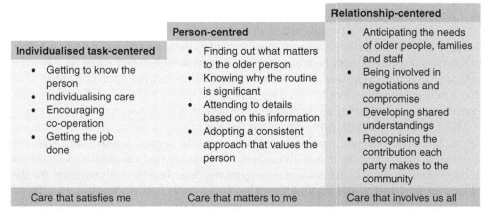

Figure 5.1 Promoting Relationships in Care Environments (PRiCE) model of quality enhancement

according to the interests of older people and families in being involved in the decision-making process and how the staff wish to promote this process.

Care that satisfies me

When staff adopted an individualised task-centred approach to care as routine practice, there was the sense that there was a high standard of clinical care given. In my study this was most regularly seen in a specialist mental health nursing home that cared for older people with complex mental and physical needs. Working in such a challenging environment meant that there was a perception that staff didn't have the time to do more than consider the physical aspects of care. Staff described a sense of reward in being able to achieve good-quality care and families described good care in terms of the physical needs being attended to.

Schneider et al. (2010) describe a similar situation in acute dementia wards, where the emotional labour involved in the job meant care workers adopted strategies focusing on the clinical aspects of care, to enable them to do the job in often complex circumstances. The language used by care workers in both my study and that of Schneider et al. (2010) demonstrate that staff see older people as individuals with likes/dislikes/preferences and try to meet these given the constraints of their workload and working environment. Although Schneider et al. (2010) conclude that this infers an understanding of the principle of person-centred care, I would suggest that individualising care still retains the focus on the task. Subsequently, the outcome is good clinical care with the consequence being that both older people and families often express satisfaction with the care they receive. This does not preclude staff from recognising details about a person's life as being important. For example, staff may report that they know about this information (see Chapter 2) but then not act on it, which means that care is unlikely to move beyond a functional approach.

Staff who tend to adopt an individualised task focus also describe motivation 'to do a good job' in terms of the clinical aspects of the job. One of the arguments I have presented in this book so far has been that the movement between different approaches to care lies in the recognition of the contribution made by older people and their families. Viewing stories shared by older people and families as a valuable contribution towards care focuses the staff perspective towards what matters to the person. This seems to complement the motivation described as 'making a difference' by staff who adopt a person-centred approach, which goes beyond providing good clinical care. So we could (re)configure staff motivation of 'doing a good job = good clinical care' as 'doing a good job = providing care that matters to the older person, which makes a difference to them'. This then becomes a mechanism by which staff might be supported in moving from adopting a task-focused approach to a person-centred approach.

Care that matters to me

In considering person-centred processes in Chapter 3, we saw how staff communicated they valued the person for who they were, rather than seeing them as a 'resident', 'patient' or 'client'. My research demonstrated the significance of stories shared by older people and their families in communicating what was important in their lives to staff. Staff who adopted a person-centred approach recognised that the details contained within these stories had the potential to make a difference and shape care in a way that 'mattered' to the older person. Families also responded very positively when these approaches were adopted as they could see that for these staff, care went beyond the physical aspects alone. Belinda Dewar (2011) used appreciative inquiry groups to actively share patient stories with staff as part of a change strategy; this supported staff in developing 'person' knowledge. Staff then developed tools to ask patients about the things that mattered to them, which meant staff were able to integrate important details into the care routines. Similarly, Brendan McCormack and Tanya McCance (2010) describe how patient stories can be organised to reflect the problem identified by the person and family as well as the solution. This approach, they contend, may result in involvement with care as well as patient wellbeing. We will be exploring some of these tools and strategies in Part 2 of this book.

Older people who experience a person-centred approach respond positively when significant details of care are included in their usual routine, as demonstrated in the practice scenario below.

Practice scenario (Brown Wilson and Davies, 2009)

I observed that one woman, who was normally chatty and engaged, was clearly withdrawn as she came into the communal area. I assumed she was having a bad day until two caregivers walked past, sat beside her and asked if they could help put her lipstick on – she visibly brightened and accepted their help. This took only a minute or so, but as the staff walked away, she was animated and engaged with those around her. When I asked the staff about this, they told me that this woman thinks she lives in a flat and that when she is coming into the lounge, she is 'going out' so she likes to have her makeup on. They told me that if they had helped her to dress, they would have helped her with her makeup before she left the room. Observing the dramatic change in this woman's demeanour clearly showed how much this detail mattered to her.

Speaking to a group of older women in another care home, I was told about the importance of time and how one of the women always had a watch on so she could tell the others the time because they could not see the clock on the wall. They told me that the staff did not understand why time was important to them, but these residents felt knowing the time gave them 'the edge' and this small detail mattered to their experience of their day. However, when we consider the outcome for older people of their experience, I also observed limitations to adopting a person-centred approach in isolation.

Focusing on the needs of individual residents, even in a person-centred way, did not always take into account the impact that decisions for one resident might have on others within the home. For example, one resident came into the lounge later than her usual time and was visibly distressed. I asked staff what had happened and they told me that they thought it would be nice if this woman had a 'lie in', as they were busy with other residents. Reorganising their time in this way allowed them to give quality time to each of the residents, which enabled a more person-centred approach. Unfortunately, this woman interpreted the change to her routine as the staff not caring about her, although they reassured her that this perception was inaccurate. While reorganising care in this way was attempting to take the residents' needs into account, it failed to involve her in the decision making, which was very different from the relationship-centred approach I observed. However, I did see opportunities taken within this same home for negotiation and compromise between staff. This suggested there were times when a relationship-centred approach was possible and indeed preferable to ensure a positive experience for the older person, staff member and those around them.

Care that involves us all

In their systematic review of the literature, Bridges et al. (2010) discuss the importance of older people and families being involved in decision making, but engaging older people in decision making remains a challenge. Ways of working collaboratively to shape the way things are done have been achieved by supporting staff to engage with patient and relative stories to inform their own perspective of caring (Dewar, 2011). This process also helped staff celebrate the positive caring process they were already engaged in, but which tended to be subsumed in concerns about targets. Working collaboratively in this way was described as a key process in meeting the expectations of patients and families (Dewar, 2011).

Language and the way information is shared may be a barrier in engaging older people in decisions. Students often describe how stories shared by older people provide important information they are able to present to practitioners when older people don't feel able to.

Practice scenario: Community

A student based in the community shared how an older woman with a terminal diagnosis missed her long walks with her husband but was told that rehabilitation is not provided in palliative care services. This student worked with the community services, the husband and wife to arrange the loan of a wheelchair that enabled the couple to share walks in the park, involving everyone in the decision-making process.

The previous practice scenario demonstrates how involving everyone in the decision-making process can support older people in maintaining social networks and feeling connected. Bridges et al. (2010) also identify the importance of maintaining existing social networks and developing new networks within acute environments of care.

Connections for older people in long-term care are similarly important but might be more difficult to maintain. Cook and Brown Wilson (2010) discuss how older people in long-term care might need support in the facilitation of existing relationships as well as in developing new relationships. When staff recognise the opportunities for social interaction between older people, they also open up possibilities for older people to make contributions to the wider community. For example, older people in my research spoke about how they 'helped' staff by not 'ringing for help' when they saw staff were busy. Older people who observed the communal routine, and were happy that this met their needs, would also accommodate the fact that sometimes their care might be delayed due to the needs of others, and so were happy to compromise when care needed to be reorganised.

For older people and families to be involved in care, it was apparent in my research that there needed to be a critical mass of staff who recognised the value of all perspectives and were prepared to engage in flexible working, negotiation and compromise. Furthermore, the person co-ordinating the care needed to adopt a relationship-centred approach that ensured everyone's needs were taken into account through the organisation of care. When staff adopted this approach, both residents and families felt able to tell staff if they needed things done differently and staff were able to support the choices of new residents as they settled into the care environment.

ACTIVITY

Consequences of different approaches to care

Return to each of the activities you have completed in each of the preceding chapters.

Identify the consequences for the older person, the families and staff when you adopted a:

- Individualised task-centred approach
- Person-centred approach
- Relationship-centred approach

Which approach provided the best outcome for the:

- Older person?
- Family?
- Staff?

Compare your answers to Table 5.2 at the end of this chapter.

Quality enhancement

Quality improvement is generally focused on activity that is measurable so that we can see the outcomes for the patient. There is considerable debate over 'nurse-sensitive' quality indicators. Nursing is considered to make little contribution to specific outcomes in the acute sector as nursing may be only one part of a wider team approach, or it may be linked to more subjective areas such as patient experience (Griffiths et al., 2008). Most of the literature around outcomes originates in the USA where researchers have access to large data sets that are linked to government funding for health care. A systematic review of 'nurse-sensitive' indicators in long-term care (Nakrem et al., 2009) revealed a complete focus on clinical care with no indicators representing the experience of older people. As we have seen from our discussion in Chapter 2, exclusive focus on the clinical aspects of care may result in the poorest experience for older people if we consider this in relation to Figure 5.1

We are beginning to see greater emphasis on the user experience in regulatory frameworks in the UK; for example, the Care Quality Commission (CQC) in England has now underpinned the importance of the service user experience as a key marker of quality (CQC, 2010). Beyond the use of patient satisfaction questionnaires or patient reported outcome measures (PROMs) there is little guidance on how to demonstrate service user experience. Our previous discussion indicates that satisfaction with clinical care might be the minimum standard we need to be considering when it comes to the experience of older people and their families in care environments. This suggests that to step up to care approaches that provide a better experience for older people, families and staff, we need to consider how we might capture this experience in ways that fit into the current quality improvement approaches in health care.

The first part of the problem is to begin to define what quality is and this in itself may be problematic. Definitions of quality may be politically driven as targets set for patient safety and efficiency influence the funding health care services receive. We all want safe and effective services that offer value for money, so the focus on these aspects of quality is important. However, exclusively focusing on technical outcomes to the exclusion of patient experience may not be the most preferable option. For example, when older people and families are asked about their care, they often refer to the relational aspects (Wilde et al., 1995; Bowers et al., 2000, 2001a; Brown Wilson et al., 2009b; Levenson, 2007; Tadd et al., 2011), although when they receive poor care, older people and their families focus on the clinical insufficiencies (Abrahams, 2011). This suggests that for older people and their families, interpersonal processes are often as important as the technical aspects.

Donabedian (1966) defined quality as measurable standards and considered how quality might be assessed in three domains: structure, process and outcome. Donabedian inferred that a good structure is likely to lead to a good process, which is likely to lead to a good outcome. By applying the discussions from the preceding chapters to Donabedian's model of quality, the care we provide might be viewed in terms of quality as shown in Figure 5.2.

Process

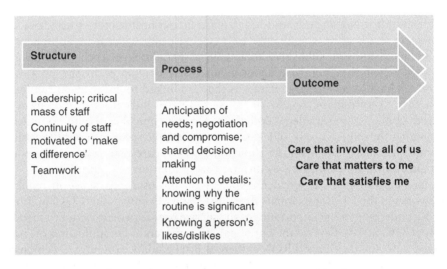

Figure 5.2   Applying Donabedian model of quality to relationships in care environments

In this book I have proposed the three approaches to care to support staff in providing good clinical care. This might start with an individualised task-centred approach, moving towards person-centred and relationship-centred approaches. The focus of our discussions has been on the process of care: what is actually done in giving care and how older people and families contribute to their care. Donabedian (1988) conceptualised the different aspects of quality as concentric circles with the inner circle being the technical and interpersonal care provided by practitioners, moving outwards to include the contribution of patients and families. Our discussions, however, have considered how the contributions made by older people and their families support engagement and participation and are integral within the interpersonal processes of care.

Donabedian (1988) contends that the technical aspects of care are given more weight because they are easier to measure compared with interpersonal processes, which need to be adapted to the individual patient. However, he also recognises that good technical care is dependent on good interpersonal processes and this is conceptualised in the individualised task-centred approach. This approach supports us in considering how the experience of older people might be linked to other indicators of quality, which is an under-explored area in nursing metrics (Griffiths et al., 2008). By considering the contribution of patients and families, Donabedian (1988) suggests the responsibility for quality in the care encounter becomes a shared endeavour. This suggests we might need to consider how the interaction between the older person, family and staff might be included as a measurement of the process in adopting the different approaches to care.

Process of care

ACTIVITY

Choose one aspect of the process of care shown in Figure 5.2 and consider how we might assess the quality of this process. Answer the following questions:

- Who is being assessed in this process?
- What are the activities being assessed?
- How are these activities supposed to be conducted?
- What are they meant to accomplish?
- How might we measure if they are successful?
- What else might be needed for this to be successful?

Structure

We have also considered the influences at work when adopting these approaches to care, which can be grouped under the structure of care. According to Donabedian (1966), structure denotes the attributes of the settings, the human resources and organisational structure. We have discussed the motivation of staff and importance of leadership for each of the approaches: individualised task-centred, person-centred and relationship-centred. We found that for the relationship-centred approach to be enacted, we needed each of these structural factors in place: leadership that enabled flexible working, and a critical mass of staff who felt comfortable in negotiation and compromise, had similar motivations and worked well as a team. What was most noticeable in our discussion on relationship-centred care was the fluidity required in adopting this approach, which makes the process difficult to define and measure.

There has been limited research on how the philosophy or motivation of care workers impacts on the process of care. Conversely, there is an established literature that underpins the importance of leadership in nursing (despite the tendency to use the terms 'management' and 'leadership' interchangeably). Although leadership from management 'sets the tone' for the care environment, leadership 'on the floor' from registered nurses and/or senior care workers is an equally important factor in how care is organised, which enables or constrains a relationship-centred approach (Brown Wilson, 2009; Patterson et al., 2011).

Ruth Anderson and colleagues have developed measurement tools for relationship-oriented leadership in care homes, which may support us in evaluating leadership that supports a relationship-centred approach (Anderson et al., 2003). Teamworking is also known to be integral to the implementation of good-quality care, with Anderson et al. (2005) suggesting that diverse interactions between staff produce a better understanding of a situation. Effective communication is a consistent element in team processes, with flexible teams noted to have communication that was open, timely and accurate in care homes (Anderson et al., 2003). This suggests we might be able to consider a range of measurement tools from some elements of the structure we have identified as influencing the different approaches to care.

Outcome

Quality outcomes tend to focus primarily on clinical indicators because outcomes in health care are often concerned with a person's health status, i.e. have we improved their health or their behaviour in any way as a result of the health care process, and are patients satisfied with the care they receive? (Donabedian, 1988). This may account for the reasoning behind the exclusive focus on outcomes in today's health and social care services. This chapter has discussed outcomes in terms of improving the experience for older people, families and staff as a result of the process of care, which is in line with Donabedian's (1988) philosophy that it is not possible to consider outcomes in isolation to the process. Patient satisfaction data is routinely collected by health and social care organisations within established mechanisms. However, there have been limited attempts in the literature to consider the patient experience in the same way. My research has mapped the consequence of care that is based on developing positive relationships to the experience of older people, families (and staff) in long-term care. However, further work is needed to define what this experience might look like in different care environments.

For the structure and process to support a good outcome, we need to establish a relationship that tells us if an attribute in the structure will influence the process in such a way as to support a good outcome. The work I have presented so far indicates the possibility that these relationships exist. I certainly saw how the structural factors we have discussed influenced the approach staff adopted, which in turn influenced the outcome for the older person, families and staff (Table 5.2).

When Donabedian (1988) speaks about relationships between structure, process and outcome, he is referring to establishing statistically significant relationships. Establishing statistical relationships between each of these areas was not the intent of my research, but my findings point to further work that will be needed if we intend to integrate the patient experience into quality improvement.

Summary

Each of the three approaches to care have consequences for older people, families and staff that can be described as:

- Care that satisfies me
- Care that matters to me
- Care that involves us all

Table 5.2   Applying the quality model

Approach to care	Structure	Process	Outcomes
Individualised task-centred	**Leadership**: Leading from the front with formal methods of communication followed up by senior care workers on the units	Communication revolves around the task at hand Making sure everyone is safe and the care is done	Making sure it is being done
	Team work: Having staff the residents don't know and who don't know the residents. Allocation by task, so all the jobs get done	Having care needs met, having to wait until staff have time to attend to me, not feeling listened to	Feeling I have done a good job, measured by tasks achieved
Person-centred	Independent working to meet resident's needs; informal pattern of communication in communal areas; sharing stories/anecdotes	Attention to important details Social conversations Changes made according to a person's needs and preferences so that what matters is captured in everyday care	Having confidence in individual staff and developing trust in them
	Having staff who know what is significant to the resident as a person Working to my strengths	Feeling valued, knowing (and trusting) individual staff to give care in a way that matters to me	Feeling I make a difference, to the individual resident when I deliver care
Relationship-centred	Leading by example with flexible and responsive patterns of working and communication; sharing stories and anecdotes Balancing perspectives of resident, family and staff	(Resident, family and staff) Organisation of care to meet needs of all residents, staff and relatives Negotiation and compromise when this is not possible; supporting relationships between residents	Feeling we are making a valued contribution to the home
	Staff who understand what is important to all of us. Negotiating workload with each other so the right person is delivering the care	Feeling valued/having confidence that I will receive care that matters to me, irrespective of who is on duty	Seeing what is important to everyone; giving care in ways that matter to the residents, because we might need care in the future

These consequences could be described as outcomes to support quality enhance-ment, using the perspectives of older people, families and staff.

Conclusion

This chapter began by making explicit the consequences for older people, families and staff when an individualised task-centred, person-centred or relationship-centred approach to care was adopted. Each of these consequences influenced the experience for each of these groups, which led to the development of a step model based on the level of participation in the decision-making process; 'care that involves us all' provided the most positive experience for older people, families and staff. We then examined how this information might improve the quality of care using the perspectives of older people, families and staff.

From the research described in this book, we have seen how the contribution of older people, families and staff influences the process of care. The level and type of contribution needs to be considered and how this might influence communication processes and the experience of care. For example, we might expect the absence of staff recognition of the contribution of older people and their families in an individualised task-centred approach and recognition and use of biographical information shared by the patient in a more person-centred approach. Subsequently, we might expect this contribution to lead to care that is described by the older person as 'care that matters to me'. We will now consider practical strategies that might support us in improving the experience of older people and their families.

PART 2

DEVELOPING
PRACTICE

INTRODUCTION

In Part 1 of this book, we examined the underpinning principles of models that focused on the task, the person and relationships when working with older people. We placed each of these models along a continuum reflecting how each supported the involvement of older people, families and staff in participating within care decisions. This continuum was based on the premise that older people, families and staff wished to be involved in decision making, although this is not always explicit within each of these models. We then considered three broad approaches that represented these models: individualised task-centred, person-centred and relationship-centred approaches. We drew on research from the acute, community and long-term care sectors, with examples of how these approaches were reflected in practice both from research and students currently working with older people. Within the chapters in Part 1 we developed an understanding of how older people and families contribute towards their care and the environment in which they find themselves. When staff recognise and value this contribution, we begin to see how we might move between different approaches to improve the experience of older people, families and staff. We concluded Part 1 with a discussion about using the perspective of older people, families and staff in making quality judgements.

Throughout Part 1, we discussed the different motivations staff had in undertaking care work. These were staff who were working in long-term care and so had made an active decision to work with older people, but we know from the wider literature that many nurses don't consider working with older people as a strategic career choice. Nurses often make decisions to work in long-term care environments due to other life factors. This is not to say they do not make an important contribution, but what my research describes is that the motivation of staff often influences the approach to care they are likely to adopt. This means that if nurses have chosen to work in an acute environment they may think that they should not need to care for older people. However, the demographic of older people that we discussed in the introduction to Part 1 means that nurses working in the acute sector will care for older people irrespective of the speciality they work in. Older people require different skills and a different approach to care than other groups of patients. If nurses feel that the acute area they work in is not an appropriate area to care for older people this may then influence their attitude toward older people and contribute towards a stereotypical view of all older people who come into their unit. Stereotyping is not exclusive to older people but it is important to be aware of the stereotypes we hold as they invariably influence our attitudes and subsequent behaviours.

MYTHS AND STEREOTYPES

Biological ageing is very noticeable to others around us as our bodies change and wrinkles appear. From an early age, we read poetry and stories where kings and rulers seek the elusive elixir of life in a bid for eternal youth. As we continuously aspire to the 'glory of youth', we expose the attendant assumption that 'age' is not something to be welcomed. This is perpetuated today in the advertising of anti-ageing formulations and reality television programmes where people strive to 'look ten years younger'. A common example is to consider how we are always impressed if an older person looks younger than our perception of their chronological age. For example, older women I know have commented on how they are treated differently in society when they have grey hair. This demonstrates that many people carry a perception of older people based on **myths** that may be perpetuated by the society in which they live. We are also exposed to myths that imbue older people with endearing qualities. While these may at first appear positive, they perpetuate a patronising image of older people as 'sweet old dears', with the underpinning assumption of a level of incompetence. We are starting to see more images of feisty older people or those who have achieved personal feats such as climbing mountains or completing extensive marathons. While these older people command our respect, this may also lead us to adopt a 'heroic' assumption about ageing, that these achievements are somehow more impressive due to a person's advanced age. These social myths circulate across our societies and as such will inform our attitudes and behaviours.

In addition, health care professionals are exposed to myths perpetuated by biological ageing such as 'incontinence is an inevitable part of the ageing process'. Biological changes means that an older person's pattern of continence will change; for example, an older person will need to void at night as their kidneys are unable to concentrate their urine, which is part of the normal ageing process. This does not invariably lead to incontinence, however if older people are in strange environments and unable to access toilet facilities they may experience an episode of incontinence. When this situation occurs, health care professionals may judge that incontinence is expected as part of the ageing process, and this may then lead to the stereotype that all older people are always incontinent.

A similar situation may occur with cognitive processing as older people process information differently and may take longer to do so. That is not to say they are not able to understand complex messages but rather may need health care professionals to adopt a different approach in their information giving. This situation may be further complicated by hearing loss, which is exacerbated in noisy environments. Health care professionals might subscribe to the myth that all older people are hard of hearing. While there are changes in the ear that are related to age, this does not inevitably mean all older people will be deaf. For those who are, often knowing when a hearing aid is required and ensuring noise in the environment is reduced will support many older people in hearing what is said to them, which is the first part of the older person being able to understand the information provided.

Myths, as I have outlined, may lead to **stereotypes** where we give a group of people the same characteristics based on personal assumptions. Stereotyping is often subconscious but invariably begins with a conscious thought. Conscious stereotyping, where we actively think about the stereotype, is quickly replaced by subconscious stereotyping, so we are not aware that we are doing it. Stereotyping is a form of categorisation – in relation to older people we consider them to be 'the elderly' and so we place everyone over a certain age into this same group. Categorising older people supports our mental organisation in a way that enables us to predict what is likely to happen. Ultimately, this is a strategy that enables us to save time and so is understandable when busy practitioners stereotype older people. However, stereotyping older people will mean that we don't always see the person as an individual or recognise the potential the older person might have in regaining their independence. This is often because practitioners are seeing older people at a point in crisis and out of their usual context. This is a particular problem for nurses who are often the gatekeepers to other professionals in the multi-disciplinary team (MDT).

This part of the book presents suggestions for using different strategies supporting the underpinning processes of the individualised task-centred, person-centred and relationship-centred approaches discussed in Part 1. We will start by considering important functional information that enables us to individualise care and so promote an older person's independence. The environment may be a key starting point in individualising care using the perspective of older people and their families. Although this could be motivated by achieving the task, i.e. in helping staff 'to get the job done', there might also be opportunities for staff to consider why this detail might be significant to the older person, thus supporting a move towards a person-centred approach. When we implement strategies, we also need a clear idea about what they are, who will be implementing them and how, and, finally, what is the intended end result. If we plan strategies with these points in mind, we can then consider how we might assess these strategies and whether they can demonstrate an improvement in the quality of care from the perspective of older people, families and staff. The strategies considered within this part have been applied in different practice contexts, including care homes, acute wards, rehabilitation services and the community.

Chapter 6 aims to support students in identifying how they might implement a biographical approach to assessment and care planning by identifying significant information shared by older people. Using a case study, we will focus on the issue of mobility and on how a biographical approach can support an older person in making decisions and overcoming their fear of falling. This chapter also presents a range of strategies that support busy professionals in identifying how they might integrate biographical information into the care planning process. A key feature of this chapter will be how we might adopt a biographical approach when caring for older people.

In Chapter 7 we will draw on environmental gerontology to explore the use of space and place for older people and how this might support us in addressing the immediate needs of all older people within the environment. Understanding the meaning of place for an older person will support us in working with them to involve them in decisions that impact on their health and quality of life irrespective of the context of care. We will use examples of supporting older people with continence and nutrition to illustrate how we might work with them to ensure they receive 'care that satisfies me'. We will consider best practice guidance developed for nurses working with older adults in the acute sector alongside what we know works in the community.

Chapter 8 considers how neighbours and friends are integral to how an older person manages their lives. Understanding the significance of such relationships is the first step in supporting older people to maintain these feelings of being connected. Being within a care environment, older people also make connections, and so recognising the potential for older people to engage with those around them is also very important. The starting point for considering social networks often lies in the questions we might ask older people, such as, if they are married, how many children they may have, where they live and the job they used to have. But stopping here means we don't really find out what the important relationships are in a person's life or how important their social network is, both to their wellbeing and to their ability to remain connected to the community in which they live. We will also consider how older people remain connected spiritually and how this might be fostered through access to the natural environment. This chapter will enable us to consider how we might provide care 'that matters to me'.

In Chapter 9 we will explore how we might recognise transitions, the impact these might have on the older person and our role as health care professionals. This may be as older people move between places including discharge planning in the acute context, supporting people to remain at home in the community and admissions to a care home. Ageing is an ongoing process and continues irrespective of where a person lives and so we will also consider how older people experience transitions while remaining in one place. We will consider how using the lens of 'transition' when caring for older people will enable us to consider 'care that involves us all'.

In Chapter 10 we will review the implementation of strategies that communicate how we actively value the contribution of older people, family and staff. We will examine how a biographical assessment might influence the outcomes of care for older people, families and staff and consider how the experience of the older person might be assessed within established quality processes.

CHAPTER 6

Using biography to plan care that matters to older people: practical strategies

Learning outcomes

By the end of this the chapter, the reader will be able to:

- Describe how a biographical approach to care planning might be conducted
- Critically examine strategies used in different care environments that promote a biographical approach to care planning
- Evaluate how these strategies might improve the care of the older person in different care contexts
- Develop practical strategies to demonstrate how care plans are shaped to provide 'care that matters to me' from the perspective of the older person

Introduction

This chapter considers what is meant by a biographical approach to care planning. We considered the evidence for using biography when supporting older people and what that might look like in Chapter 3. Biographical methods are discussed in some detail in the research literature, but provide limited guidance in how such information might be gathered and used in busy practice environments. There are many opportunities for 'therapeutic encounters' as an older person is supported with personal hygiene or nutritional needs. It is at these times that health and social care practitioners exchange personal information, enabling the older person to develop a sense of trust. Many students tell me of similar situations they experience where important information is shared with them as they are perceived to be 'less' busy than registered nurses. I would term these therapeutic opportunities 'spontaneous encounters' as they emanate from other activities. These encounters are useful in busy environments where there is often limited time to sit with individuals to undertake a life history. Such encounters can be helpful in shaping a picture of the older person and what is important to them. However, it is rare that students are able to relate how they integrate this information into the usual care planning process. Therefore, we should also consider how we might develop a more strategic approach to involve the older person in the care planning process through biographical assessment.

This chapter provides a pragmatic approach in how we might move from the 'spontaneous encounter' model of obtaining biographical information to a more structured approach where all staff have access to relevant information that may impact on care decisions. These care decisions may have a long-term impact on the older person, and so should take into account significant information shared by older people. This chapter considers a number of strategies developed through research and practice that might promote a biographical approach to care planning. Although different, each strategy has similar underpinning factors that lend themselves to a biographical approach to the care planning process by:

- Supporting the professional in engaging with the personal perspective of the older person
- Eliciting significant details about a person's life or opening up the opportunity to consider significant details at a later point
- Fostering communication strategies that respect and value the perspective of the older person
- Developing personal and responsive relationships between staff and the older person

The strategies presented in this chapter are those that fit particularly well with the person-centred approach presented in Chapter 3. They can be used to move from accessing a person's preferences or likes/dislikes to finding out what matters to them in their care and their life. The strategies presented here have been used in practice and are intended as a starting point in the implementation of a biographical approach in your area of practice. We will integrate a biographical approach into the usual assessment process, using this approach to get to know the older person and to inform clinical judgements, ensuring 'what matters' to the older person is captured and transferred into everyday care.

Finding out what matters through the assessment process

Often the person being admitted to a care environment will be assessed by the nurse verbally and the written assessment will be completed away from the person with the nurse identifying relevant goals for treatment. These may take into account information that the older person has shared and the nurse may then discuss this treatment plan with the older person. I would suggest this approach limits the participation of older people in decision making; they have been consulted but they are not really involved in the decision-making process. To involve patients in the decision-making process, staff in Belinda Dewar's (2011) study developed a series of questions they asked each patient on admission to find out what mattered to them (Box 6.1). Although patients were surprised to be asked these questions on admission, the patients who responded felt they could then approach nurses with subsequent information further into their admission.

Box 6.1   The 'all about me' framework

- What would you like staff to call you?
- How would you feel if staff use terms like 'darling', 'love', 'honey' when they speak to you?
- Who are the people closest to you and who do you want us to communicate with?
- What are your thoughts and feelings about being in hospital?
- What is your understanding of why you are in hospital?
- Is there anything that is worrying you about being in hospital?
- Is there anyone you would like to speak to? (doctor, chaplain, family member, friend, neighbour)
- What is important to you while you are in hospital?
- What support do you need from the people that care for you?

Dewar (2011: 219)

In many health care environments in the UK, the nursing assessment is based on the activities of living (ALs) defined by Roper, Logan and Tierney in the 1980s (Roper et al., 2001). This approach provides a useful framework to explore the abilities of a person before they required the care they now need. This might be related to a deterioration based on an existing health condition or due to an accident. Assessing the abilities of an older person prior to the current episode of care supports the nurse in understanding the immediate needs of the person as well as considering future goals. The list of ALs (Table 6.1) promotes an assessment of the whole person: physical and emotional issues, spiritual needs and the opportunity for the person to raise concerns over death and dying. We will be using this table to consider how we might develop our assessment using biographical information using a case study throughout this chapter. How such tools are used will be down to the skill of the individual nurse doing the assessment. In my own practice, I have often seen issues such as spirituality, sexuality or death and dying ignored as irrelevant when assessing older people. Adopting a biographical approach to care planning will support us in understanding the meaning of ALs from the perspective of the older person.

Using the case study of Dorothy, we will use Table 6.1 to consider how the information Dorothy shares with us might be relevant to our assessment. This exercise will support us in using the ALs to get to know the older person so they might share their aspirations and goals, not only for their treatment but also their future.

Table 6.1 Activities of living

Activities of living	Dorothy's biographical information
Maintaining a safe environment	
Communicating	
Breathing	
Eating and drinking	
Eliminating	
Personal cleansing and dressing	
Controlling body temperature	
Mobilising	
Working and playing	
Expressing sexuality	
Sleeping	
Death and dying	

Adapted from Roper et al. (2001)

Case study: Dorothy Brown

Dorothy Brown is 88 years old and lives alone in a rural part of the UK. Dorothy married late in life and had no children; she is now widowed. Dorothy is being admitted for a knee replacement and so this would identify Dorothy's key problem as her mobility. Thus we might need to find out what her mobility was like before she came in. To this question, Dorothy generally answers that her walking wasn't very good as her knee was always 'giving way', that's why she is 'here'. Dorothy might share that she lives near the farm where she grew up, which grazes cattle and sheep. Living on the farm until she was married, she has always been active, although she feels she has slowed down as she has aged. Dorothy has always owned dogs and she currently has a Jack Russell whom she walks twice a day over this farmland, which is notoriously difficult to walk over with potholes and uneven surfaces that the cows have churned up. She might tell you that her dog is a 'rabbiter', so she needs to take him where there are rabbits for him to chase. She can sometimes feel breathless if she has had a good walk with him, but within her house she has no breathing difficulties. Walking in general has become increasingly difficult as her knee has deteriorated but this is a key feature of her daily routine. She is paying her friend to look after her dog while she is in hospital.

Assessing Mobility

ACTIVITY

Using Table 6.1 write down Dorothy's key problems for her mobility.

- What is Dorothy's usual pattern of mobility?
- What implications might this have for Dorothy's treatment?

Physical activity is important for all older people and supporting older people to increase their physical activity can improve conditions such as heart disease and chronic obstructive pulmonary disease, as well as reduce bone loss. Indeed the evidence suggests that after 10–12 weeks of regular strength or aerobic training, the 'clock' can be turned back by nearly 20 years in relation to muscle strength and aerobic fitness, even when exercise is started later in life (Skelton et al., 2011). Exercises that improve strength, gait and balance are known to improve postural stability and prevent falls (Skelton et al., 2005). Nurses and other health care professionals may subscribe to the common myth that increasing age and frailty make exercise unnecessary or too dangerous, but the evidence suggests that sedentary behaviour is the real risk with advancing age (Skelton et al., 2011).

Case study: Dorothy Brown (continued)

Dorothy lives alone in her bungalow which she tries to keep in good repair with the help of a local tradesman. She has recently asked Age UK to come and fit modifications such as grab rails and outdoor steps so that she can remain independent even with reduced mobility. Dorothy is unable to do very much in the house as she feels dizzy when she looks above her shoulder height, so her nephew who visits regularly helps with 'odd jobs' when he visits. She has some help from the village, with a local woman coming in to help her with the housework once a week. This woman has recently moved to the village with young children and is unable to drive, so Dorothy has helped her by driving her and the children shopping when this was needed. Dorothy also has another friend who helps her do things around the garden. She has local gardeners to do the lawns and manage the fruit trees in what was called 'the orchard'. Dorothy and her husband built their bungalow on the orchard of their previous property and although she has arranged the garden to be as low maintenance as possible with shrubs, she still likes to have pots with pansies and herbs that she can manage herself. She has been finding it difficult to manage the watering with her knee but finds this inability frustrating.

Maintaining a safe environment

- What do we know about Dorothy's environment and her approach to risk?
- How will this support planning for Dorothy's discharge?

ACTIVITY

As people age, they are more likely to experience a range of different conditions that, put together, are described as geriatric syndromes. Geriatric syndromes might include loss of mobility, falls, hearing/vision impairment and if not treated may lead to increasing frailty and poor outcomes (Inouye et al., 2007). Frailty has also been described as an accumulation of deficits across multiple physiological systems (Rockwood et al., 2006), but there is no agreed definition. Frailty is characterised by the older person's diminished resistance to physiological stressors, making an older person more vulnerable to adverse outcomes (Ferrucci et al., 2004). The involvement of more than one system means there is a cumulative effect which is why the greater the degree of frailty, the more an older person is at risk of poor outcomes such as increased falls, delirium or pressure sores. If we reduce the deficits that contribute to frailty, such as reversing muscle weakness and improving nutrition for example, we might be able to reduce the impact of frailty for the older person.

Case study: Dorothy Brown (continued)

Dorothy slipped on the drive in the snow as she was 'tidying things up'. This fall has now made her very cautious as she doesn't want to fall again. Luckily she had her emergency call pendant, which she activated and one of her neighbours came to help. This has focused Dorothy's mind on the importance of being independent as her sister had Parkinson's disease and lived in a nursing home until her death. Dorothy may tell you that she has no children to support her, which places her more at risk of needing a nursing home if she loses her independence. This has motivated Dorothy to look after her health and remain as fit and active as possible.

If older people present to hospital with a fall it is good practice to undertake a falls risk assessment and then consider a multi-factorial intervention (National Collaborating Centre for Nursing and Supportive Care, 2004). There have been many systematic reviews considering the issue of falls in hospitals. Bridges et al. (2009) reviewed the evidence and found that clinical judgement was as good as using a falls risk assessment tool, and exercises that focus on improving balance and gait were found to be effective. Good practice suggests that when older people present as having a fall in the last year, there should be an in-depth assessment of what led up to the fall, which leads to a person-centred plan that reflects the patient's goals and aspirations. This should also include a medication review (Hartikainen et al., 2007) and a referral to the physiotherapist/falls team for further assessment and intervention (Bridges et al., 2009). While in many places, this might be standard practice, we should be careful of making judgements without considering the older person's perspective. One man nursed by a student was quite angry to find that he had the words 'falls risk' in red written above his bed. No one had discussed his fall with him and he felt this had been a one-off occurrence and was not relevant to his current admission. Involving this gentleman more in the decisions surrounding his care and speaking with him in more detail about his fall might have improved his experience of this admission.

Mobility can often lead to issues in getting to the toilet on time, particularly for older women, so we might use this to lead on to a conversation about elimination by asking how they manage getting to and from the toilet and where this is located at home. Retaining continence is an important aspect of care for many older people and Dorothy is no exception. There may sometimes be the assumption that incontinence comes with age and we will consider this assumption and the impact on older people in the following chapter.

Case study: Dorothy Brown (continued)

Dorothy tends to suffer from cystitis, which is an issue that she has managed for many years by having a structure to the amount of and types of drinks she has over the course of the day. Most importantly, Dorothy might share at this point that she only has decaffeinated drinks. This is particularly important as it prevents the over-stimulation of her bladder. Another issue that Dorothy may share is that she generally wakes up to use the toilet once or twice each night. For this she will need access to a close bathroom so she can find her way independently as she does not want to bother anyone. Dorothy also ensures she maintains a regular pattern of daily bowel actions.

Elimination

- How might Dorothy's elimination be affected by her hospitalisation?
- What might be the concerns for Dorothy?
- What practical strategies might you employ to alleviate these concerns?

ACTIVITY

Earlier we suggested that frailty was characterised by an older person having diminished physiological reserves, making it more difficult for them to cope with stressors. Hospitalisation may create a number of stressors for older people, such as changes to their usual routine, which may include what they eat and drink. At home, Dorothy eats well and tries to drink little and often between meals. Knowing how older people maintain their nutrition prior to coming into hospital will provide valuable information in ensuring the food and drink provided meet their requirements and preferences. We will be considering this in more depth in the following chapter.

Case study: Dorothy Brown (continued)

Dorothy's mealtimes remain synchronised to the farming clock and she likes to eat fresh food, although she needs to be careful in what she eats due to her gastric reflux. Adopting a biographical approach, we might think to ask at this point how she does her shopping, to find that Dorothy needs to be able to drive into the local town a few miles away as there is no village shop where she lives. Coming from a farming community, Dorothy does not believe in the use of supermarkets and she buys what she needs from the farmers' market every Saturday to support the local farming community. This has issues for how far she might have to walk in the high street as parking can be difficult, even with a disabled badge.

ACTIVITY

Eating and drinking

- What routines might it be helpful for Dorothy to maintain while in hospital?
- What are some of the key issues for Dorothy when she is discharged?
- What might place Dorothy at risk of malnutrition?

Adopting a biographical approach is equally, if not more, important in long-term care with older people, staff and families. The importance of choice is now being recognised as an area for further development (Simmons et al., 2011). In my research, the assessment process in care homes that adopted a relationship-centred approach would help reveal the important details in care routines and then consider how these could be adopted to ensure everyone received care using a person-centred approach (Brown Wilson and Davies, 2009).

Case study: Dorothy Brown (continued)

Adopting a biographical approach, we might make a key observation that Dorothy wears a wig and looks very smart, wearing simple makeup. We might tactfully ask her why she wears a wig and she would share that she lost all her hair when she was young. She wears a wrap on her head when she is unable to wear her wig and discloses that she does not like people to see her without this. We are now getting the sense that Dorothy has always been an independent woman and we might assume this with her personal hygiene. Dorothy has a shower and prefers this at night but she is willing to accept help if this aids retaining her independence. Dorothy is used to being busy and will find an enforced period of rest difficult. Dorothy may recollect at this point how she and her sister had to hide their steaming coffee mugs and quickly turn off the radio when their father came around the corner. To this day, she finds it difficult to sit down, although she recognises that age seems to be slowing her down. As you notice her appearance, you might ask her if she has anyone special in her life and she will tell you that her husband died some years ago from Parkinson's disease but she still misses him terribly. Dorothy was his main carer and felt very depressed after his death, isolating herself from her usual activities and networks. She realises this was not a good thing to do but her approach to life now is to take every opportunity!

Personal hygiene needs and sexuality

- How are Dorothy's personal hygiene needs and sexuality linked?
- What are the key routines that Dorothy needs to maintain while in hospital?
- What support might Dorothy need on discharge?
- What are the important issues for the community team when Dorothy returns home?

Ensuring attention to details such as the ones described by Dorothy are taken into account requires nurses to be more active in seeing the whole person and what this means to the care encounter. This might require different ways of organising work to ensure nurses are more visible and are perceived by older people to have time to listen to them. Using caring conversations as described by Belinda Dewar (2011) might be a way to support nurses in considering how to reconnect with patients (Box 6.2). This requires a level of courage and a preparedness to negotiate when perspectives differ (Dewar, 2011). As mentioned in the first part of this book, this approach often required others in the care environment to support this process.

Asking if Dorothy has anyone special in her life would be an example of how a caring conversation might begin. This starts with curiosity but requires both courage and compassion as you are letting Dorothy know that you are prepared to speak with her about intimate relationships. We are going to look at intimate relationships in more detail in Chapter 8. Having elicited Dorothy's feeling about her late husband, this might lead us to ask if she has any concerns in relation to death and dying.

Case study: Dorothy Brown (continued)

We might ask Dorothy where her husband was buried and she will tell you about the family graves she has at the local village church and how she looks after them. This requires her to wash the gravestones and place plants or flowers on the graves, and she has asked a friend to do this for her while she is away. She has attended this village church all her life and remains an active member of the faith community. She finds going to church on Sunday begins her week well and she supports all the social events of the church.

Dorothy was recently asked to open the church fête, and she will tell you how the fête was the highlight of her year as a child. She would take her pony and give pony rides when she was younger and then ran the 'bottle stall' as she got older. She remembers her father taking a pig and greasing its tail; if any of the villagers were able to catch it, they could take the pig home. This was always great fun to watch. We might see from this story that spirituality for Dorothy is about helping others in the community as well as going to church. When she was able, Dorothy would visit friends in the community who were dying, she would help people do their washing or do some cooking for them. Now that she is unable to do these things, she finds it difficult to always accept help from others knowing that she is unable to reciprocate. She is still able to support an older friend who appears to be having memory problems by ringing her in advance of church engagements and collecting her in the car to drive her to events outside the village.

Table 6.2 Attributes of appreciative caring conversation

Key attribute	Dimensions	Key questions/statements that support the attribute in action
Being courageous	Courage to ask questions and hear responses. Trying things out. Feeling brave to take a risk.	What matters? Help me to understand why you have done that. What would happen if we gave this a go?
Connecting emotionally	Inviting people to share how they are feeling. Noticing how you are feeling and sharing this.	How did this make you feel? I feel … You made a difference to my day because …
Being curious	Asking curious questions about even the smallest of happenings. Looking for the other side of something that's said, and checking things out.	What strikes you about this? Help me to understand what is happening here. What prompted you to act in this way? What helped this to happen? What stopped you acting in the way you would have wanted to?
Being collaborative	Talking together, involving people in decisions, bringing people on board, and developing a shared responsibility for actions. Constantly checking out with others if your interpretation is accurate; looking for the good in others to encourage participation and collaboration.	How can we work together to make this happen? What do you need to help you to make this happen? How would you like to be involved? How would you like me to be involved? What would the desired goal/success look like for you?
Considering other perspectives	Creating space to hear about another perspective. Recognising that we are not necessarily the expert. Checking out assumptions. Being open and real about expectations. Recognising that other perspectives may not be the same as yours and feeling comfortable to discuss this in an open way.	Help me to understand where you are coming from. What do others think? What matters to you? What do you expect to happen while you are here? What is real and possible? What would it look like if we did nothing?
Compromising	Working hard to suspend judgement and working with the idea of neutrality. Helping the person to articulate what they need and want and share what is possible. Talking together about ways in which we can get the best experience for all.	What is important to you? What would you like to happen here? How can we work together to make this happen? What do you feel you can do to help us to get there? What would you like me to do?
Celebrating	Making a point of noticing what works well. Explicitly saying what works well and asking questions that get at 'the way'. Continually striving to reframe language in the affirmative.	What worked well here? Why did it work well? How can we help this to happen more of the time? If we had everything we needed, what would be the ideal way to achieve this? What are our strengths in being able to achieve this? What is currently happening that we can draw on? I like when you …

ACTIVITY

Death and dying

- Do you think Dorothy would find it difficult to speak about dying?
- What might be her key concerns as she moves towards this transition?
- What might be Dorothy's wishes for future care?
- How might we document this?

A biographical approach is concerned with how an older person approaches their life and the goals and aspirations they might have. This will provide an opportunity to understand how older people wish to be involved in the decision-making process. Just because they are ill does not mean older people wish decisions to be made for them. However, a US study found that nurses often made assessments on whether or not to ambulate a patient based on their previous experience of older patients (Doherty-King and Bowers, 2011). The evidence suggests that older people can lose up to 40 per cent of muscle strength after three weeks of immobilisation (Skelton et al., 2011), but Doherty-King and Bowers (2011) found that it was often not until the patient was being prepared for discharge that nurses focused on the loss of function. At this stage, many older people may then require additional community-based resources.

As busy practitioners, we can sometimes place our own expectations on what an older person of a certain age should expect from treatment. This might mean when an older person such as Dorothy exceeds our expectations, we then consider that further treatment is not required. In doing this we miss what is important to the older person.

Case study: Dorothy Brown (continued)

Dorothy shares her love of swimming with us. In fact, we learn that she represented her Women's Institute at a county competition for her freestyle swimming. She tells us that when she was on the way to the competition, she was told that she would be in the 50+ group which made her very apprehensive as she was then in her 70s. Her fears proved groundless as she won first prize! Dorothy now feels her swimming days are over as her recent falls mean she lacks confidence in going up the stairs of the local swimming pool. When asked, she tells you she would like to return to swimming. This now becomes a further long-term goal and can be addressed by structured hydrotherapy sessions overseen by a physiotherapist to assess the progress of her knee.

Long-term mobility

- What are the implications of this information for Dorothy's plan of care?
- What referrals might be made and why are they important?

ACTIVITY

Adopting a biographical approach suggests that while Dorothy doesn't mind asking for help to retain her independence, she feels uncomfortable asking for too much support when she can't reciprocate. This leads us to consider the importance to Dorothy in being able to drive, for which she will need good mobility. This might lead us to find out whether alternative treatments such as hydrotherapy might be used to improve Dorothy's muscle strength, ensuring she could get back to driving as soon as possible. Dorothy wishes to return home as quickly as possible but lives alone and so will need a period of intermediate care to continue mobilisation. On returning home, Dorothy will also require support from the community re-ablement team and may benefit from seeing the falls team to reduce her fear of falling.

As Dorothy has her knee operation and is supported with her personal hygiene, some of these stories might have been shared informally with different members of staff. This is often the case, with different members of staff then acting in isolation on this information. This means that receiving person-centred care will be dependent upon which members of staff are on duty. This results in what I would term an 'ad hoc' biographical approach, and often the students I discuss this approach with will tell me that this information is shared with them routinely. Often this information supports the development of personal and responsive relationships, but it might not then be used to attend to significant details in the care plan. The question now is how we might adopt a more structured approach and use this information to ensure the care that is delivered is consistent across all staff and all shifts. The previous part took you through a skilled approach to the use of ALs. By developing a conversational approach and asking some structured questions at the beginning of the assessment process, more detailed information might be used to develop an appropriate care pathway with key biographical information. We will now consider how the stories Dorothy has shared with us might be distilled into her care planning.

ACTIVITY

Review your assessment of Dorothy

- Consider whether this assessment differs from others you might be conducting in practice – what are the key differences?
- How might you develop your practice to include biographical assessments?

In a review of the literature, McKeown and colleagues (2006) found that interventions that used life-story work were generally undertaken to improve care by understanding the person and maintaining their identity. However, creating a life-story book, for example, can be time-consuming and does not always result in changes to care (McKeown et al., 2006). Moos and Bjorn (2006) suggest that to be effective, life-story interventions should also include translation of the life story into care interactions and actively encouraging residents in meaningful activity. The 'Who am I' document developed by the Alzheimer's Society also enables staff to identify who the person is, and the significant routines they might have, to provide an in-depth understanding that may result in improved outcomes for older people in acute settings. It is important when caring for people with dementia that we don't assume they are unable to tell us what the problem is or what matters to them. Different people will be at different stages in their dementia and may well have different levels of recognition and memory function. It is important that nurses have a greater understanding of what dementia is and how it affects individuals. Adopting a conversational style using the biographical approach, to assessment, as we did with Dorothy, would be appropriate to engage people with mild to moderate dementia in a discussion about what mattered to them. Allowing them time to talk about their memories supports an improved understanding about what might stimulate different types of behaviour. This can support staff to enable people with dementia to remain engaged with the care being provided rather than resisting what they don't understand.

In Dorothy, we are beginning to see a picture of an independent woman who is used to physical activity rather than a frail older woman of 88 years. This might lead us to discuss Dorothy's key goals and consider how we might manage these both in the short and longer term.

Case study: Dorothy Brown (continued)

The key issues that Dorothy raised in terms of her priorities would be:

1   To regain her independence as soon as possible by being able to drive again
2   To be able to walk her dog across uneven fields
3   To reduce her fear of falling

These are long-term goals that are important for Dorothy, which we might share with the wider multi-disciplinary team. We might then identify the best way to approach them while Dorothy is in hospital and then once she returns home. Issues that are important to Dorothy in the short term would be:

1   To retain her independence in her personal hygiene
2   To support her continence needs with reduced mobility
3   To maintain her safety in hospital and avoid a fall
4   To undertake a medication review
5   To support Dorothy's religious routine
6   To explore the issue of advance care planning with Dorothy in more detail

---

Dorothy's perspective provides a challenge for nurses and other professionals as this is different to the perspective many professionals might adopt. Recognising Dorothy's perspective is the first step in supporting her to achieve these goals. Adopting a biographical approach to assessment develops a clearer picture of the person Dorothy is and the life experiences that have shaped her. There is no one way to achieve this; what is necessary is that there is a process whereby older people feel comfortable in telling nurses their concerns.

Summary

- A biographical approach enables the perspective of the older person to be recognised
- Finding out what matters is an integral part of a biographical approach to assessment
- Considering significant details in a person's life will support the care planning process
- Developing conversational strategies is a mechanism to engage the older person in the decision-making process

Conclusion

Throughout this chapter, we have considered strategies that support a biographical approach to assessment and care planning. These strategies enable us to develop a picture of what the older person values, allowing us to understand how they manage their life, their health and the goals they may have for their current period of ill health. This is particularly relevant when considering how to support older people in living an active lifestyle to reduce the risk of conditions that might lead to increasing frailty and poor outcomes. This chapter highlighted how using the biographical approach enables the older person to identify goals and aspirations that challenge our assumptions as professionals. We will continue this theme in the following chapter.

Further reading

Skelton, D., McAloon, M. and Gray, L. (2011) 'Promoting physical activity with older people', in Tolson, D., Booth, J. and Schofield, I. (eds), *Evidence Informed Nursing with Older People*. Oxford: Wiley Blackwell.

Tolson, D., Booth, J. and Schofield, I. (2011) 'Principles of gerontological nursing', in Tolson, D., Booth, J. and Schofield, I. (eds), *Evidence Informed Nursing with Older People*. Oxford: Wiley Blackwell.

Tolson, D., Day, T. and Booth, J. (2011) 'Age related hearing problems', in Tolson, D., Booth, J. and Schofield, I. (eds), *Evidence Informed Nursing with Older People*. Oxford: Wiley Blackwell.

CHAPTER 7

Understanding interactions between the person and the environment

Learning outcomes

By the end of this the chapter, the reader will be able to:

- Describe how the environment influences the health and wellbeing of the older person
- Critically examine strategies that might be used in different care environments that promote a positive person–environment interaction
- Evaluate how these strategies might improve the care of the older person in different care contexts
- Develop practical strategies to demonstrate how care plans might support person–environment interactions

Introduction

Considering the interaction between the environment and older people, this chapter draws on the wider literature to consider the importance of place on three levels: the physical environment, how spaces and places are used on a social level (the social environment) and how older people attribute the environment with meaning through interaction (psychological environment). Peace et al. (2011) describe the concept of 'options recognition' when older people recognise they may need to make decisions about their environment. Options recognition occurs when changes occur within each of the physical, social and psychological environments. This is especially valid in health and social care as many older people may be accessing services that could impact on the environment in which they live at a point of crisis. This may include relocation or, alternatively, it may include the re-configuring of the social environment within the home environment recognising the importance of this for the older person and their families.

Understanding the meaning of place for an older person will support us in working with older people to involve them in decisions that impact on their health and quality of life irrespective of the context of care. Home is more than the building in which we live. Although our 'home' may be the focal point for this, there will also be factors in the local community which will give us a sense of home. This information is significant if we are supporting older people in moving from their homes to other forms of housing as home may also be about the familiarity of the wider community. A biographical approach may support us in understanding the meaning of home for an older person. If we are supporting older people to remain in their own homes for longer, as practitioners we may need to consider issues such as the functional limitations imposed by the building or what we might consider to be barriers to enabling the older person to continue to live in that building. However, if we consider the perspective of 'place' as described in environmental gerontology, we begin to understand that for the older person, it is not the amount of barriers but rather the magnitude of these barriers and how these barriers impact on the usability of the environment (Nygren et al., 2007). The usability of the environment within an older person's home supports the continuation of meaningful daily routines that impact on wellbeing. Feeling 'in control' within the environment has been seen to be influential across a number of European countries (Iwarsson et al., 2007).

In this chapter, we will consider the meaning of 'place', the impact of environmental barriers, the usability of the environment and the ability of the older person to control their environment as a framework to guide our discussions. While there are many measures that can be used to consider these issues in detail, we will take a more pragmatic approach and consider how we might use these concepts to inform our practice when caring for older people in a range of different environments. We will start by considering some of the environmental barriers that might inhibit 'care that satisfies me' from the perspective of the older person.

Physical environment: addressing environmental barriers

Hospitals are often focused on the needs of acutely ill patients, providing care often at times of crisis; so these environments need to deliver safe and effective health care. In the UK, successive governments have worked to ensure hospitals meet targets that demonstrate they are providing safe and effective health care. The NHS is funded by the taxpayer and so hospitals are accountable for how the money is spent. This has led to a target-driven culture to reduce, for example, death rates, infection rates and waiting times. This means the public are better informed about the quality of the health care they are receiving and that the money being spent on health care is providing them with good-quality health care. A (potentially unforeseen) consequence of this has been that the focus on these targets has removed some of the focus from the patient experience. An interesting example of this is the reduction of waiting times for operations such as joint replacements. This focus on getting things done quickly has meant that the acute environment might not always be the most appropriate environment for caring for the older person, who might require additional time for rehabilitation before being discharged home. This has meant the additional time spent on caring for an older person might be seen as not appropriate for an environment that is tasked to achieve a certain amount of operations to maintain waiting lists.

This may have contributed towards nurses falling back on stereotypes of older people as portrayed in the media and wider society to help them organise their workload more effectively. The work undertaken by my students has challenged these stereotypes and, in some cases, demonstrated that it is possible to provide more person-centred care without taking additional time.

Practice scenario: Surgical unit

Following a hip replacement, staff insisted that Mr Peters should use continence aids which he was unhappy with. The student spoke with Mr Peters and found that he only had a short distance to walk to the toilet at home, which he managed with a Zimmer frame. The student arranged for his bed to be moved closer to the toilet and liaised with a physiotherapist to provide him with a Zimmer frame so that Mr Peters was able to mobilise independently to the toilet. This return to independence increased his wellbeing.

There have been times when supporting older people with dementia or communication problems might take more time, but equally this time has been saved at a later date when problems were avoided using this information. The evidence drawn on in the following sections is derived from best practice statements developed through a systematic review of the literature (Bridges et al., 2009). The practice scenarios are provided by students who identified some of the barriers and solutions when implementing best practice guidance.

One of the biggest myths is that incontinence is caused by age. While there are age-related changes to the urinary tract, this does not necessarily need to result in incontinence. However, when there are co-morbid conditions and increasing medications, this may increase the likelihood of incontinence as people age. This does not mean that incontinence is a normal consequence of ageing. What it does mean is that there will be additional needs for the older person to support their continence, as discussed in the previous practice scenario. Indeed, best practice suggests that all older people should find the toilet facilities accessible, which also includes good signage for those with sight problems (Bridges et al., 2009). When students have spoken to older women who have experienced incontinence, these women discuss how they manage their continence but are unable to do so in a busy ward environment, which then results in incontinence as the next scenario suggests.

Practice scenario: Surgical unit

Mrs Smith needed surgery for a fractured wrist following a fall at home and was immediately assumed to be at risk of falls. When she was found walking to the toilet unescorted, she was stopped and asked to return to bed. This delay caused incontinence and so she was given an incontinence pad to wear. Mrs Smith became increasingly withdrawn from staff and family.

Wayfinding might be particularly challenging in the acute sector as it is not always clear where toilets are located and many of the bays and corridors in modern wards look very similar. Students in seminars I have led describe how they asked families to bring in something that is recognisable to the older person to put beside their bed to assist with finding their way back to the right bay. The reflective glare of ward lights and shiny surfaces, including floors, also pose challenges to older people, particularly those living with dementia. A colleague told me about a person with dementia who due to the shine on the bluish floor tiles was convinced her bed was in a pool of water, and so did not want to get out of bed. Involving the older person in the assessment of the problem (in this case refusal to get out of bed) is crucial if we are going to move beyond our own professional assumptions. This is further exacerbated by the clutter of corridors with little design consideration given to how the older person might negotiate these barriers. Even in outpatient clinics, the environment can be difficult to negotiate and thus become disabling for the older person.

Another concerning issue is that when older people become incontinent, they are seldom offered support to regain that continence through referrals to specialist nurses. There is substantial evidence that specialist nurse intervention increases continence in stroke patients (Thomas et al., 2008). Booth et al. (2009) suggest that up to 70 per cent of urinary incontinence can be treated or ameliorated but in spite of this, nurses rarely refer older people to specialist services. When nurses subscribe to the stereotype that all older people are incontinent, it means that continence will not be discussed and subsequently the older person's needs will not be identified, referrals are not made and specialist support is not accessed.

ACTIVITY

Consider an older person with continence problems

- What questions might you now include in the assessment process?
- How might this person's biography influence the care plan?
- What changes could you make to the physical environment to promote continence with older people?

What we have discussed so far is an inadvertent lack of understanding of the needs of older people through the application of stereotypes. However, in their study about dignity in acute hospitals in the UK, Tadd et al. (2011) report nurses telling patients that if they are unable to use the commode at the bedside, then they must 'do it in the bed', resulting in a loss of dignity for that person. With an increasing emphasis on safety within health and social care, guidance will be provided across an organisation to prevent that accident happening again. While we do not know which trust was being referred to in Tadd et al.'s (2011) study, we might infer that a person could have fallen from a commode when being transported to the toilet, and so transporting people using commodes was no longer permitted. The interpretation of this guidance that the only alternative was for the older person to soil their bed is clearly not acceptable. This requires a wider discussion of ward practice and the consideration of other options in how people are assisted to go to the toilet. This is not an uncommon problem, with nurses describing how they struggle to put person-centred care into practice on busy wards due to competing priorities (Bradbury-Jones et al., 2011).

There are times when older people may present to acute services with delirium as a result of infection, which may be (but not exclusively) in the urinary tract. Delirium is a condition that presents with acute confusion where multi-component interventions such as promoting safety, hydration, maintaining fluid/electrolyte balance and oxygenation may ameliorate symptoms (Milisen et al., 2005). This treatment may also be difficult as people experiencing delirium may not be as rational as usual and understanding a person's background may be the key to instituting treatment. There is sparse evidence on the efficacy of interventions to prevent delirium or interventions that reduce length of hospital stay (Siddiqui et al., 2007). We know that starting antibiotics immediately for urinary tract infections (UTIs) improves the person's condition more quickly (Turner et al., 2010) and a routine screen for UTIs may detect potential causes of delirium. However, there may be times when such a simple diagnosis might be missed if nurses think that all the older people they see have dementia and then put their behaviour down to a diagnosis of dementia rather than delirium. There is a particularly high risk of this when older people come through medical assessment units, where there is a focus on speed to move the person through to a ward environment. Families may identify that their relative does not usually have memory problems or behave in this way, but busy nurses using stereotypes to sort their workload may not give this piece of information the credibility it deserves. At this point, the potential diagnosis of delirium is delayed and so might be missed until the condition worsens, by which time the length of stay has been increased.

If we consider these examples alongside the principles of relationship-centred care in Chapter 4, we might think about how the 'anticipation of needs' might help us find a solution to these complex issues. In Chapter 4, we considered how we drew on the perspectives of older people, families and staff to find a solution that may have involved negotiation and compromise. First, let's consider whose perspective is dominant in these situations: we might consider that the examples above are a direct result of the needs of the organisation becoming overwhelming for nurses, so that nurses working in the acute sector are unable to consider any of the other competing needs. We have just discussed how continence needs are important from the older person's perspective.

Undertake the following activity to consider how the perspective of the older person and that of the staff (and organisation) might be brought further into alignment.

Return to the example from the previous activity

- Using your biographical knowledge of this person, how might you anticipate this person's continence needs?
- How might you organise care taking this information into consideration?
- Are negotiation and compromise required and if so, how might they be achieved?

Patient satisfaction (care that satisfies me) is an important area of quality for the organisation, with the needs of the older person now seen to be as important as the needs of the organisation. Recognising that issues such as continence will become a recurring issue in an increasingly ageing population might lead us to consider how we could (re)manage the ward environment so the issue is not seen as problematic. This means the focus has now moved to the environment and how this can support older people's needs. This may remove the concern that many nurses have that older people's needs are not suited to an acute environment. Ensuring the older person receives good clinical care may require negotiation and compromise with staff, other patients and families, as we reorganise care to meet the needs of everyone in the care environment.

Incontinence is often a factor that precipitates admission to a care home (Bridges et al., 2009), which may perpetuate the ongoing stereotype that incontinence comes with age. Organisation of care in many care homes tends to revolve around the issues of managing incontinence, which may precipitate people being taken to toilets en masse prior to mealtimes. While it is important to ensure incontinence is managed appropriately, it is also important that we don't bypass those older people who retain their continence. The routines older people adopt when living in care homes may enable their continence but as with the acute sector, the environment and working practices of staff may also disable this ability, which will reduce over time. This is particularly difficult when people are not able to move independently.

Practice scenario: Care home (Brown Wilson, 2007)

Freda had a stroke and was unable to mobilise independently. Retaining her continence was of particular importance as a stroke had left her with few other abilities. One team of staff recognised the importance of this and would ensure they organised their morning so that three staff could be with Freda shortly after coffee time when they knew she would require the toilet. There were times when things might not have gone according to plan and on these occasions, staff re-negotiated their workload

(Continued)

(Continued)

with other staff, and where necessary with other residents, to ensure they were able to be at the assigned point for this toileting procedure. This went beyond 'care that satisfies me' to 'care that matters to me'.

For older people who continue to live in their own homes, we also need to ensure they are supported to retain their continence and consider strategies within the home environment that enable them to achieve this. This may be focused on self-care strategies that enable them to identify problems with continence, not as a result of their 'old age' but that may be due to infection, lack of hydration or related to nutritional intake. As with the previous discussion in the acute sector, it is of equal importance to refer older people for specialist advice for incontinence, rather than simply managing the incontinence. Strategies that promote continence also need to consider how older people undertake activities that give their lives meaning and a biographical approach to care for older people is an important step towards this.

The usability of the environment (social environment)

Another area that has been the focus of older people receiving poor care has concerned nutritional intake. The *Hungry to be Heard* report (Age Concern, 2006) demonstrated that in the UK many older people were coming out of hospital more malnourished than when they were admitted. While there is some evidence to suggest this may be addressed in part through the use of supplements (National Institute for Health and Clinical Excellence [NICE], 2006), there still remains an issue with older people being supported at mealtimes.

Practice scenario: Medical ward (Tadd et al., 2011)

One older woman has been given her meal and tries very hard to eat it. After a few mouthfuls she gives up. The catering assistant who comes to take her plate away notices she hasn't eaten very much and makes a comment that she mustn't be hungry today. The situation goes unnoticed by the nursing staff.

This is not an isolated situation, with students reporting that even with protected mealtimes older people who require support are not receiving this, until their meals have gone cold. While we may be concerned that there are insufficient staff to work around each person individually, perhaps on these occasions we need to think more creatively about how mealtimes might be organised within a ward environment to promote a more social occasion for those who may need assistance. While there is a move to reduce social spaces in ward environments due to pressure on bed space, students also report the use of social spaces as additional storage rather than being used to support people having their meals in a different space from where they spend the rest of their day.

Consider an older person who might require additional support with mealtimes

- What do you know about this person's approach to mealtimes before this episode of care?
- Is there any information you could use to improve this person's intake?
- What changes might you make to the social environment at mealtimes?

Supporting older people to move to a dining space promotes mobility and interest, which in turn may promote appetite. Recognising the importance of meals for older people moves beyond knowing preferences in diet (although this is still important) to understanding how social interaction might enable people to engage with their meals in a different way. Being on hand to observe when people are having difficulty and so supporting them when needed, is of great value.

The protected mealtime initiative in the UK has stimulated wards to reconfigure space differently, and there are many examples of good practice in promoting nutrition and hydration in older people (National Patient Safety Agency, 2009). The mealtime as a social occasion is now acceptable practice in care homes with a range of good practices being implemented.

Practice scenario: Care homes (SHINE Project)

One team chose to try a new dinner time routine in one of its units. The problem was that residents were coming into the kitchen and this made mealtimes hard to control. The team planned to have a trial where all residents would be seated in the dining room, asked for their choices of food and provided with a waited service. They found that this was a lot less stressful for both the staff and the residents and that the residents were eating their meals a lot better than before. Before rolling this idea out to the rest of the home, they identified that a lot of the residents were changing their minds when they saw the plated up food. In order to avoid wastage, the home is now creating an illustrated menu to show residents the choices for each day.

Although it is widely accepted that nutrition scoring tools support the monitoring of nutrition in at-risk older adults (Elia and Russell, 2009), there is no accepted approach to nutritional assessment that is consistently used across care homes. This is very different from the US system of care homes, where monthly assessment of older people across quality domains such as nutrition, falls, pressure sores, etc. are collected as part of the national funding system. Care homes in the UK are run by many independent companies, with each company operating their own system of monitoring clinical care such as nutrition. In 2007, a large survey for the British Association for Parenteral and Enteral Nutrition (BAPEN) (Elia and Russell, 2007) suggested that 45 per cent of people admitted from care homes were malnourished and a recent regional survey of care homes found that 1:3 older people were still at risk of malnutrition, with 42 per cent of older people being identified as malnourished in that sample (Norris et al., 2011). This suggests that nutrition remains an ongoing challenge in care homes as it does in hospitals.

Nieuwenhuizen et al. (2010) undertook a systematic review of interventions in older adults and found that the greatest body of evidence was for the implementation of oral supplementation. Oral supplementation has been recommended as the first line in combating malnutrition in older adults (NICE, 2006). This guidance does not take into account the range of factors impacting on the nutritional intake of older people in institutions such as hospitals and care homes (Table 7.1).

Table 7.1 Factors influencing the nutrition of older people

Physical factors	Large meals are often overwhelming to the older person; offer small servings
	Provide high nutrient snacks at regular intervals
Sensory factors	Combat loss of taste perception by developing food with richer tastes
	Enable older people to smell the cooking of food to increase appetite
Social factors	Ensure a suitable environmental ambience

From Nieuwenhuizen et al. (2010).

Practice scenario: Protected mealtimes across one hospital (McClelland, 2007)

Before the implementation of protected mealtimes, 11 out of 45 patients experienced an interruption during mealtimes. During the protected mealtime trial in 2007, this was reduced to four out of six patients. Of these four interruptions, only one was unavoidable, and two patients did not specify the reason. From this trial it was concluded that protected mealtimes were successful and improved the patient experience. Following this trial, 10 acute medical, and department of medicine for the elderly, wards had successfully implemented protected mealtimes.

The previous practice scenario reflects experience from practice where 'space' is used differently by reconceptualising mealtimes as a social time rather than as a further clinical task. This is similar to intervention studies that suggest improving the environmental ambience was sufficient in itself to improve nutritional intake (Nieuwenhuizen et al., 2010). Such evidence should prompt us to examine how we might reconfigure the ward space to provide a sense of 'place' at mealtimes, promoting social interaction within the ward environment. This might require us to think differently about the use of staff and the use of volunteers to facilitate different ways of managing mealtimes. In a review of the literature on nutrition in hospitals, Kubrak and Jensen (2007) recommend that nurses need to take more responsibility for nutritional intake in hospitals through assistance and recording, and they suggest future studies are needed to understand the barriers to effective nutritional care in hospitals.

Implementing a biographical approach is the first step in finding out what matters to older people, and we have seen how we might use this to improve clinical care. Understanding how an older person approaches their life will also provide insight into how independent they wish to be at mealtimes. Knowing this might stimulate us to consider specialist referral and support, involving occupational therapists in the assessment process. This will ensure we provide older people with the tools they require that enable them to remain independent in their nutritional intake. We need to understand the role of hydration for older people, and providing easily accessible water at the correct temperature is the first step in this (Royal College of Nursing, 2007). However, we also need to ensure older people are able to reach, pour and drink this water. Occupational therapists can assess these activities and provide the right equipment to facilitate this process. There may also be times when hydration is important for the older person and the support required by the older person may need to be prioritised over other activities. This may be of particular significance when supporting people with dementia and/or delirium.

Dehydration might prompt confusion states that are not usual for an older person. Identifying this early sign and prioritising hydration may reduce the length of stay someone has in hospital as prolonged dehydration may lead to further complications in the person's health status, which may be avoidable. We have already read about examples where staff prioritised these activities knowing their significance to the older person and using biographical information to engage the person with this process, while they were receiving the support they needed. Adopting a biographical approach may be the first step in identifying different ways of reconfiguring mealtimes in different environments.

Nutrition may pose different problems as older people 'age in place' in the community; with current cohorts of older people having lived through years of war and rationing, which may still influence how they shop and cook. Many older people remember the time before 'sell-by' dates were used, and so these dates may not have the same meaning they have to professionals who are concerned with their 'duty of care'. Older people living alone may struggle with mealtimes as 'cooking for one' might be substantially different from previous roles they may have had within the family as they cooked for many. Understanding the implications of these aspects of their biography is important in terms of the social support that older people might access.

There are now a number of services that older people can access and pay for, where a hot meal is delivered each day, but whether people eat these meals is another matter. A further issue for older people in the community lies in the use of restricted diets such as low-sodium, low-cholesterol and low-sugar diets. In a prospective, randomised controlled trial, Zeanandin and colleagues (2012) found that these diets resulted in low nutritional intakes in people over 75 years, with many societies not providing guidance for supporting those older people with renal conditions, heart disease or diabetes.

The meaning of 'place' (psychological environment)

I have structured this chapter around the different types of environment identified in the literature. We have covered the physical and social environments and we now move on to the psychological environment. This section will focus on how older people perceive their environment, most notably the concept of 'home'. As this section progresses, it will become clear that the boundaries between each of these environments can blur, as we consider the concept of home and the competing perspectives this raises. This is particularly evident when we consider the international health policy of 'Active Ageing', where older people are encouraged to be independent and remain active participants within society (Brown Wilson, 2011). Active Ageing (WHO, 2002) is being implemented in many countries using the concept of 'ageing in place', where retirement communities, both in the USA (Shippee, 2009) and Australia (Cheek et al., 2007), have been developed providing increasing levels of care within the same area by the same organisation. The ageing in place concept enables older people to move between services while remaining within the same community. This suggests that the notion of 'ageing in place' is more than simply considering the home in isolation. The concept of 'ageing in place' remains widely defined but it is not a static principle, as older people redefine and renegotiate their associations with 'place' (Andrews et al., 2007).

It may be helpful at this point to consider the notion of 'place' from the perspective of environmental geography. In this discipline, there are similar but competing notions of 'place' and 'space' that may be of value to health care professionals. At this point, I am drawing on the work of Janine Wiles and colleagues who have explored the concept of 'place' as a process as it relates to older people. In her 2005 paper, Wiles outlines the nuanced difference between the notion of 'space' referring to universal and abstract ideas such as geometrical distance, while 'place' is a smaller part of the overall space that is experienced by a person, holds meaning and shapes the social relationships between people. In this way, places are not only shaped by people, but places also shape people and the society in which they live (Wiles, 2005). However, places are often seen as a 'context' for either living or indeed health care, rather than as a 'place' to live. An example of this might be providing health care in a person's home. While health professionals might be concerned with the space in which a person lives, they might not always be aware of the impact the reinterpretation of home as a medicalised environment may have on the social processes, not only for the older person, but also for the entire family.

Practice scenario: Community

Joe was receiving palliative care at home and, as he deteriorated, it was suggested he required a hospital bed in the living room. His wife resisted this and subsequently became labelled as 'difficult' and not 'caring' for the needs of her husband. As the student undertook a biographical assessment with Joe and his wife, it became clear that for this couple, the intimacy of lying together at night and being able to cuddle was very important and something they did not want to lose as Joe approached the end of his life.

In this practice scenario, the staff only saw the difficulty of climbing the stairs. In this way, the house was seen simply as a 'space' that was not conducive to the needs of their patient. How the decision to use a hospital bed might impact on the social use of the home or the relationship of that couple was not considered. This example demonstrates how different perspectives of 'place' need to be negotiated and understood from beyond the health care perspective.

'Place' is often associated with a person's life history, creating a sense of attachment through associations with events, activities and treasured memories (Andrews et al., 2007), but older people themselves may see the concepts of 'place' and 'home' as very different. In a New Zealand study, Wiles and colleagues (2012) asked older people about their understanding of 'ageing in place' and found differing perspectives: some older people spoke about being attached to physical spaces such as homes or gardens, while others spoke about connections to people in the area. There was also the distinction between house and neighbourhood, where some older people might consider moving 'house' as it was becoming difficult to manage, but wished to remain in the neighbourhood, close to the social connections they had made. How older people reach decisions to move might be understood by considering the work of Sheila Peace and colleagues (2011), who suggest that the interplay between these different factors causes older people to consider different options in relation to their living arrangements. They term this 'options recognition' where older people consider the physical, social and psychological environments and realise that things are changing.

ACTIVITY

Recognising the options open to older people

Think of an older person you have known in either a personal or professional capacity who needed to move.

- List the factors that you thought were important in prompting the move
- List the factors family members thought were important in prompting the move
- List the factors the older person thought were important

What were the similarities and differences between the lists? Which priorities won and why do you think this was? Keep this work, as we will be returning to this same person in coming chapters.

Peace and colleagues (2011) suggest that older people may consider their own physical capacity, in relationship to the different level of their environment. This means they might consider their interest in maintaining their physical environment alongside the meaning this environment has both on a social and psychological level. Environment, however, is not simply restricted to the immediate home in which people live but extends to the wider community, which may be perceived by older people as a resource enabling them to retain independence and autonomy through access and familiarity (Wiles et al., 2012). In the UK, a study for the Joseph Rowntree Foundation certainly found that many older people actively managed their lives and seized opportunities to live what they considered 'a good life'. This may have been in the face of concomitant losses, but it demonstrates the importance of being part of a community and an inter-dependence where people look out for each other and provide support according to their abilities (Godfrey et al., 2004). For many older people, the ability to age in place will also be influenced by the physical, personal and emotional resources they have at their disposal, and this will be different according to the resources of the communities in which an older person lives (Godfrey et al., 2004; Wiles et al., 2012). Such factors as these are integral to older people being able to age successfully as the case study of Dorothy Brown demonstrates.

Case study: Dorothy Brown (continued)

Dorothy speaks about her love of riding that she has had throughout her life. She explains how she had to give up riding due to a health condition and so spent 25 years working for 'Riding for the Disabled'. Once this was no longer possible, Dorothy still retained her interest in horse riding by following the local hunt until problems with her knees prevented her involvement. Now Dorothy's health prevents her from physically pursuing these activities she maintains her interest in these areas by subscribing to the *Horse and Hound*. She shares these magazines with friends and so is able to speak about shared interests when they visit.

This discussion highlights the importance of understanding the concept of 'place' from the perspective of the older person, which is underpinned by the importance of a biographical approach if we are to consider how best to support older people to 'age in place'. However, for some older people, remaining in their own homes will not always be possible, either due to a lack of family or community support, or due to a health condition that creates needs for which there are inadequate community-based resources. In their review of the geographical gerontology literature, Andrews and colleagues (2007) concluded that it was becoming more accepted that it is better for older people to be cared for in 'home-like' environments if they are unable to continue to live at home. This is somewhat problematic, as the concept of 'home' means different things to different people who live in care homes, as it does to those living in the community.

In care homes, some older people told me that they had begun to feel like it was their home as they were able to maintain relationships with friends external to the home or retain links with places near the home, including the natural environment. One older woman described how she chose the home as it held memories of places she used to visit with her husband and enabled her to have access to the outdoors, of which she was particularly fond. For these older people, it was about connections to people and places in the wider community. For other residents, developing this sense of 'home' can be problematic, as the meaning of a person's home may be tied to shared memories with family and friends and activities they may no longer be able to do. My research suggests that it may be of greater benefit to consider care homes as communities where everyone has a role to play (Brown Wilson, 2009; Brown Wilson et al., 2009b).

Practice scenario: Care home (Brown Wilson, 2007)

Ann-Marie had come to work in the care home later in life, following a redundancy in her previous job. Her motivation was 'to give something back' to society. She told me that it was important for her to make older people feel as 'special' as they would in their own home. This meant that if there was something they needed to help them feel comfortable, that as they would in their own home, then she would make the effort to do it for them.

Subsequently I have worked with staff caring for people living with dementia. People living with dementia are often unable to recognise the care environment as 'their home'. These staff considered ways they could support the person with dementia to feel comfortable by playing music they recognised, having familiar artefacts such as knitting patterns or magazines to look through or supporting them to put 'their feet up', as they might in their own home (Brown Wilson et al., 2012). This suggests that understanding the meaning of place from the perspective of the older person can support staff in identifying meaningful activity for older people relevant to their interests and abilities. If we consider that everyone has a role in the wider community of a care home, this may be the first step in making people feel 'comfortable' in what is essentially a communal environment. Using a biographical approach can identify activities that an older person might consider 'meaningful', which would ensure people felt they had a valued role to play within the wider community.

Disabling environments restrict older people from engaging in activities they enjoy and a study undertaken by Judith Torrington at the University of Sheffield demonstrated how many care homes tended to design towards safety. Under-utilisation of areas in care homes for meaningful activity, particularly outdoor areas, can have a detrimental effect on the quality of life of the older person (Torrington, 2007). Older people living in care homes probably do not receive what would be considered the minimum requirement of fresh air and natural light, particularly in the winter months (Gilliard and Marshall, 2012). We will return to this issue in more depth in the next chapter where we consider how older people remain feeling connected.

Summary

Promoting 'care that satisfies me' involves:

- Adopting a biographical approach to care, which identifies what is important for older people and helps to overcome some of the more common stereotypes of ageing
- Considering good clinical care in context to the environment in which care is being delivered
- Recognising that the use of physical space can have disabling effects on older people who may struggle to maintain their continence and nutritional intakes at times of health crises or when continuing care is needed
- Understanding that the 'place' of care also has social and psychological implications for older people

Conclusion

Throughout this chapter, we have considered strategies focusing on how care might be delivered, taking into account the different environments: physical, social and psychological. We considered how the perspective of the older person might shape care, given the constraints of the physical environments of health and social care. The different examples were underpinned by suggestions for rethinking how we see the environment using a biographical approach. This has been particularly relevant when considering the social element of the environments we work in and how this might improve some of the practical aspects of supporting older people. We concluded with a discussion about the importance of 'place', which has particular relevance when supporting older people in long-term care. This discussion highlighted the importance of 'place' as a process which shapes the way people live and the relationships they engage in. We will continue this theme in Chapter 9 when we focus on transitions.

Further reading

Booth, J. (2011) 'Continence management', in Reed, J., Clarke, C. and McFarlane, A. (eds), *Nursing Older People: A Textbook for Nurses*. Buckingham: Open University Press.

Booth, J., Kumilen, S. and Zang, Y. (2011) 'Promoting urinary continence', in Tolson, D., Booth, J. and Schofield, I. (eds), *Evidence Informed Nursing with Older People*. Oxford: Wiley Blackwell.

Dickinson, A. (2011) 'Nutrition including food preparation', in Reed, J., Clarke, C. and McFarlane, A. (eds), *Nursing Older People: A Textbook for Nurses*. Buckingham: Open University Press.

Jackson, J. and Polding-Clyde, S. (2011) 'Promoting nutrition with frail older people', in Tolson, D., Booth, J. and Schofield, I. (eds), *Evidence Informed Nursing with Older People*. Oxford: Wiley Blackwell.

CHAPTER 8

Understanding how older people maintain connections with those around them

Learning outcomes

By the end of this the chapter, the reader will be able to:

- Describe how a biographical approach might support the social and intimate relationships of the older person
- Consider how feeling connected to people, places and nature may promote emotional and spiritual wellbeing in older people
- Critically examine the barriers and facilitators in different care environments that support older people in maintaining connections that hold significance for them
- Develop practical strategies that enable older people to maintain connections with those important to them and develop relationships with those around them

Introduction

The previous two chapters have focused on important issues of physical health that contribute to the geriatric syndrome and increase the risk of frailty. This chapter will focus on issues surrounding emotional wellbeing that impact on an older person's mental health. I am using the term connections as this encompasses how we relate to people, pets and places, as well as to a higher force, whether that be God, nature or the universe. Feeling connected to the people we come into contact with every day is important, as are the relationships we develop with pets and places. These may sometimes have a greater impact on our emotional, social and spiritual wellbeing. When we begin to speak about these issues, we begin to charter uncomfortable waters as this often requires an emotional connection with those we care for. Irrespective of which care environment we work in, this emotional labour often goes unrecognised and is rarely part of the quality system. However, we know that when older people speak about quality of care, they often refer to relationships.

Relationships are important to all of us; we live in relationship throughout our lives and this does not alter as we age. Relationships enable us to feel connected to places and people around us. These connections will mean different things to different people. For some, significant relationships may be focused on families while for others, they are those in their immediate neighbourhoods. Relationships may also be developed across our life span with different relationships assuming importance at different times in our lives. Social ties and networks may alter as we age but the importance of relationships does not. What constitutes significant relationships will differ between people and we will use this chapter to explore how a biographical approach might support us in finding out what matters to the older person and those around them.

We will consider how the social connections of older people are relevant in different contexts and the part this might play in our assessment and care planning. We know that social networks can influence health and wellbeing and we will discuss how the different typologies of social networks might support us in considering the social support older people might have available to them. We will also consider how older people themselves see their social support and this may alter depending on how often older people have contact with those in their social network. Health professionals tend to consider social support in terms of families and next of kin, when this might not always be the case. We will consider how a biographical approach might support us in suspending our own assumptions about what might constitute significant relationships for the older person. As we age, maintaining significant relationships may become more difficult but not impossible and this is true of intimate and sexual relationships as well. There are many myths surrounding sexuality in old age and we will explore how we might use a biographical approach to consider what is important to older people in this area of their lives and how this might become part of the assessment and care planning process.

Connections may also be about places and considering the importance of community ties and having access to nature. We will consider spirituality in its widest sense of understanding who we are and how we are in relationship with the world around us, considering practical ways of supporting older people to maintain important connections that give them a sense of who they are and how they fit into the wider world.

Being connected to those around you

Relationships are a key feature of how older people describe their care experiences. In a systematic review of the qualitative literature of acute experiences of health care, Bridges and colleagues (2010) found that a reciprocal relationship with staff meant that older people and their families felt reassured that their needs would be met and that they were valued as a person. In long-term care environments, my research suggests that older people and families actively engage with staff to develop relationships and look for ways of contributing towards their own care (Brown Wilson et al., 2009b). Supporting people in the community is also about developing relationships with staff, but staff also find they may be supporting existing relationships between the older person and those close to them (Clissett, 2007).

The common feature across these care contexts is the importance older people and their families place on developing relationships with those around them. Belinda Dewar (2011) speaks about the importance of family and patients feeling connected with what is happening and how this can be facilitated by staff asking what families think and using language that is understood. Certainly, many students in seminars I facilitate speak of scenarios where older people have withdrawn from involvement in care and consider how a biographical approach can reconnect them with what is going on around them. This can be as simple as finding out what is important to the older person and implementing this in their care.

In their model of person-centred nursing, Brendan McCormack and Tanya McCance (2010) describe the 'sympathetic presence' of the nurse as being beside a person in their experience of health care. Here the nurse acknowledges their inability to fully understand the experience from the person's perspective but respects their feelings and expresses that they are there to support that person during the experience. 'Sympathetic presence' is quite an abstract term, but has been interpreted by students I work with as spending time listening to the person, acknowledging their concerns and negotiating changes to the care plan that demonstrate that these concerns have been heard.

Relationships with staff often mean the difference between a good day and a not so good day. In one project in which I was involved, older people were asked to write down their experiences of care using creative writing techniques (Brown Wilson et al., 2011). Supported by a professional writer, a group of women described their experiences using metaphors. One woman wrote of her experience that 'the best care was like sunshine, warming your back through a thin blouse' (p. 13). While these experiences were in long-term care, Wadensten et al. (2005) describe a similar pattern in acute environments where morning conversations set the tone for the remainder of the day. Tadd et al. (2011) also describe how the language used by nurses in hospital wards, such as 'dear', 'sweetheart' and 'babe', reduces the opportunity for further discussion as older people feel they and their opinions are not being respected. Bridges et al. (2010) suggest that for patients and carers in the acute sector, feeling connected by feeling they are respected and welcomed, helps reduce feelings of anxiety.

Knowing the staff caring for you is important for older people. Ensuring older people know a little bit about you is an important part of the reciprocal nature of the relationship. Sharing personal information needs to be considered in the context of the relationship being developed and the context of care – telling an older person the details of a night out might not be an appropriate disclosure but speaking about a common interest that you might have with an older person or their family member might be. Developing personal relationships like this facilitate the feelings of mutual trust older people may have in you, that may then enable them to disclose personal information of a sensitive nature.

Practice scenario: Care home (Brown Wilson, 2007)

A son told me how two of the care workers had gone to the school where his father had taught. As they got talking, it transpired that one of the care workers had been taught by his father. This gave the family a sense of connection with the staff.

Molony and colleagues (2011) found that older people were able to develop social relationships with staff and other older people following a move to smaller group homes compared with usual nursing homes. In this study, older people described their ability to come and go, make contributions to life in the home, and freedom to engage in social and meaningful relationships (Molony et al., 2011). Janine Wiles (2005) suggests that health care needs to promote communities of care that support older people in retaining their independence and autonomy in ways that are flexible and sensitive to difference, recognising the importance of building and maintaining relationships, when in receipt of care services.

Recognising important social relationships

ACTIVITY

In the final activity in Chapter 7, you considered an older person whom you knew (either on a professional or personal level). Now with reference to this same person:

- List the important relationships in this person's life before they were considering their move
- Are any of these relationships intimate?
- List the important relationships following their move
- How might the move impact on these intimate relationships?
- Look at the lists before and after the move – how do they differ and why do you think this is?

Older people also need to feel connected to others around them who are not staff, such as other patients on a ward or other residents and families in long-term care. Communal environments, whether they are in acute or long-term care, provide opportunities for relationships with those in close proximity, which also means opportunities for contributions to be made. It is important for older people to feel comfortable where they are staying, whether this is an acute ward, an intermediate care environment or a care home. Patterson et al. (2011) identify the importance of a sense of security for older people, particularly in relation to single-sex accommodation; knowing neighbours in the same bay may also be important for many older people. This may be similar to the experiences of older people in long-term care, where staff are not always aware of the relationships older people may develop within a care home or the impact sensory impairment may have on developing relationships (Cook et al., 2006).

Staff seeing opportunities for the development of relationships between older people is the first step in supporting them to feel connected, which may be as simple as recognising when older people have something in common and then considering how this relationship might be facilitated (Brown Wilson and Davies, 2009). We have seen from examples in previous chapters how groups of older people support each other, making a contribution to the wider community; such examples included information giving or being able to tell others the time. It must also be recognised that not all older people will want to make these connections with those around them, with some not willing to invest effort into what they believe to be transitory relationships (Brown Wilson et al., 2009a). This is different from older people withdrawing from relationships with other older people due to sensory loss such as difficulties with hearing and/or vision (Cook et al., 2006). The importance of hearing loss affecting how older people can be engaged in their care has been outlined in previous chapters and these are not dissimilar issues for older people engaging in relationships with others around them.

Feeling connected to those closest to you

Many of us will have had someone with whom we have become very attached spending much of our time in their company, or in close proximity. Attachment is considered important to an older person's sense of physical and mental wellbeing, contributing a level of security that enables them to confidently interact with their environment (Cookman, 2005). If we see older age as a period of decline, we are less able to consider the issues of intimacy and sexuality as the assumption is these issues become less important with age. Our approach towards sexuality in older people is often governed by the social rules and expectations of the society in which we live. If we consider the issue of ageing in Western culture, the ageing body is not considered something of beauty, with women in particular targeted by advertising to remain youthful in order to be attractive. Older men who express sexual intent may be labelled as behaving in an inappropriate or lecherous way (McAuliffe et al., 2012), as this is one of many stereotypes about sexuality (WHO, 2010). Sexuality with older people is often limited to sexual expressions where it is often considered inappropriate for older people to engage in sexual activity, particularly those with dementia or those who are not heterosexual (Ward et al., 2005). For those who have spent many years of their lives together, there may be a lifetime of sharing a bed and feeling someone close by, and this need for intimacy, closeness and touch does not necessarily decline with age (McAuliffe et al., 2012). Ill health and chronic conditions may impact on an older person's ability to maintain their intimate and sexual relationships, which can have an impact on the wellbeing of the couple, particularly when a partner goes into a care environment (McAuliffe et al., 2012).

Sexuality is expressed in many ways, including how we present ourselves, how we dress and what we do. Older people in care environments may require support to express themselves in these ways, as demonstrated in the following practice scenario.

Practice scenario: Care home (Brown Wilson 2007)

I noticed Andrea asking Freda what she intended to wear that morning and then place two necklaces against the dress so Freda could decide which matched the best. When I asked about this later, Andrea told me that she knew Freda's son was visiting today and she always liked to look her best, so it was important that her jewellery matched her outfit as wearing nice jewellery had always been an important part of Freda's life.

Understanding the significance of these details following a biographical approach ensures a more person-centred focus. When staff focus exclusively on tasks, details such as makeup and jewellery may not always be seen as a priority. This is compounded by the fact that we may not see older people as capable of sexual expression, which is another myth of sexuality and older age. Older people, including those with dementia, are capable of sexual expression, with some studies describing flirtatious behaviour between residents (Hubbard et al., 2003). Sexual expression such as this is often considered inappropriate in care settings, with such behaviour seen as problematic (Ward et al., 2005). In a chapter written with colleagues, we recount a situation where an older woman and man developed a relationship while in hospital and by chance ended up being admitted to the same care home. It became clear within the home that this couple wished to develop an intimate relationship, which challenged both staff and family. However, this relationship was facilitated by staff enabling the couple to sleep in the same room, which afforded privacy to maintain their relationship (Brown Wilson et al., 2009a).

For many older people, retaining sexual activity is important. For some this may be focused on intimacy, while for others this may also include penetrative sex (Gott and Hinchcliffe, 2003). Not recognising that older people may be engaged in sexual relationships places them at risk of sexual health problems (Gott, 2005), as demonstrated in the following scenario.

Practice scenario: Medical unit

A man was admitted with genito-urinary problems for which they could find no cause. The student had developed a trusting relationship with this gentlemen by undertaking a biographical assessment, where he disclosed he was having casual sex and it was found that he had chlamydia and he was discharged following treatment.

It is important we do not make assumptions, treating all older people as a homogeneous group or basing our assumptions upon chronological age. Adopting a biographical approach supports the development of relationships between older people and staff that enable older people to feel comfortable in raising sensitive subjects such as sexuality. Older people themselves may not raise these issues as they may be concerned about the response of staff because of their age.

Practice scenario: Surgical unit

Mrs Taylor was worried about resuming sexual relations with her partner following her operation, but didn't like to ask because she felt that having sex might be considered inappropriate at her age. The student didn't feel able to answer her concerns and so asked a more senior colleague with whom Mrs Taylor felt comfortable. Mrs Taylor was able to disclose the difficulty she was having in undertaking her sexual relationship and given appropriate post-operative advice to help her resume this important part of her life.

In Chapter 6 we considered how we might take a biographical approach to assessment and one of the suggestions I made was to ask if there was anyone 'special' or close' in the person's life. For Dorothy, this enabled her to speak about her feelings for her husband who had died, but equally, it might have created an opportunity for older people to speak about their partners, who may be of the same sex or long-standing friends with whom there is an intimate relationship. We might follow this by asking if they have any concerns in respect to this relationship (or the absence of this relationship), which creates an opportunity to disclose worries or concerns about sexuality or sexual expression. This is very different from asking about next of kin, which may not be a partner or friend. In recognising a person's sexual expression, we are enabling them to express who they are in every aspect of their life, and it is important particularly in residential environments that we support older people in sexual expression, whether this is by supporting intimate relationships or attending to significant details of appearance. We must also recognise that places are shaped by but also shape the way in which people relate to one another, on an intimate as well as broader scale, and this has implications for health care (Wiles, 2005).

When we become unwell, we often want people we know and who know us close by. Bridges et al. (2010) found that maintaining connections with those close to the person was one of the interventions that helped relieve anxiety for patients and carers during periods of acute health care. We all feel vulnerable when we are unwell, so feeling connected to those who are closest to us is also important.

Recognising social networks

Return to the person in the activity at the beginning of this chapter:

- Draw a circle with a picture of the person in the middle
- Now draw consecutive circles, keeping the person in the middle
- Starting from the closest circle and moving outwards, write the names of people most important to the older person in the closest circles, with those less important as the circles move outwards
- What support might the person need to keep in touch with each part of their network?

This is a description of their social network. In the following section there are two typologies of social networks (see Box 8.1):

- Choose the appropriate typology for where the person lives and describe the main features of their social network
- What are the implications for this person?
- What social support might this person need as they age and how might this be provided?

From the previous activity, we can see that social networks and social support are different. Social networks provide the structure we might need when we require social support. Consider who you turn to with everyday problems and how this might differ from those you turn to with life-changing issues, for example. This demonstrates how different parts of our social network provide different levels of support at different times in life. In the community, feelings of social connection have been linked to increased health and wellbeing (Stephens et al., 2011). However, socio-economic status, ethnicity and gender are part of the social context in which we are connected through our network of relationships. In New Zealand, where a bicultural society exists, Stephens and colleagues (2011) found these factors had a negative impact on the perception of social support among the Maori population, which are known to be disadvantaged when compared with white New Zealanders. In Canada, the importance of family ties was more important where there was lower socio-economic status due to industrial decline compared with more affluent areas where community life was the most salient issue (Zunzunegui et al., 2004). It is thought that socio-economic status may outweigh other protective factors that social support has in communities with large community and family networks (Stephens et al., 2011).

Clare Wenger has developed a typology of community-based networks (Box 8.1) and suggests that a locally integrated network of family, friends and neighbours reduces the risk of depression for older people. However, there are different strengths and weaknesses for each of these networks with different implications for the provision of services (Wenger and Tucker, 2002).

Box 8.1   Typology of community-based networks

1 *Local family dependent support network* – is focused on close family ties, few neighbours and peripheral friends
2 *Locally integrated support network* – includes close relationships with local family, friends and neighbours
3 *Local self-contained support network* – typically has arms-length relationships or infrequent contact with at least one relative but the primary reliance is on neighbours
4 *Wider community-focused support network* – has an absence of nearby relatives but active relationships with distant relatives, usually children, and a high level of friends
5 *Private restricted support network* – is associated with an absence of local kin, few nearby friends and low levels of community contacts

From Wenger and Tucker (2002).

Understanding an older person's social network may also be of value when considering the implication for social support, whether this is from the hospital or community. For example, an older person might have a large social network including family and friends, but have a low perception of support. This may be due to the number of contacts older people have on a daily basis (Cornwell, 2011), as social contact is necessary for older people to feel connected with and supported by their social network (Stephens et al., 2011). As people age, their social networks may reduce as a result of life transitions including relocation or retirement, the experience of illness, the impact of chronic conditions and the death of contemporaries. This may mean that the social networks of older people may reduce, along with the level of support they receive from these networks. This places many older people at risk of social isolation. Asking people about their perceptions of loneliness and isolation may be a useful way to capture some of the effects of lack of social support and poor social networks (Stephens et al., 2011).

Loneliness and isolation are not confined to living within the community but might also be experienced by older people in care homes. In early work by Bethan Powers (1991), a typology of relationships between older people in care homes was also developed (Box 8.2), with balanced networks that included family, friends and staff showing a greater sense of connectedness. Maintaining these connections may be difficult for older people as they enter care homes at a higher level of dependency than previously. This means that maintaining connections both within and beyond the home may require more support from staff.

Box 8.2 Typology of residents' social networks in care homes

- *Institution-centred networks* – consisted of ties which were simple, concentrated on the institution and were of low intensity
- *Small cluster networks* – contained established cliques of residents operating within larger networks. These residents regularly spent time together, providing opportunities for reciprocity and support
- *Kin-centred networks* – concentrated on relationships with family who visited regularly. Residents in these networks often resisted forming relationships with other residents based on fear or the disturbing behaviour of others
- *Balanced networks* – had the largest amount of people within them, drawn from contacts that included other residents, staff and families. These networks showed the greatest interconnectedness within the home

After Powers (1991).

Maintaining connections

Being connected to large networks is a recent yet increasingly common phenomenon with the advent of social and professional networking sites. People, young and old alike, are using social media as a mechanism to stay connected with those around them and the wider world. Technology is largely responsible for this, with computers, smartphones and iPads now making such networks increasingly accessible. Families may also be dispersed geographically, including overseas, and so maintaining contact becomes increasingly important.

Practice scenario: Care home

Staff in a care home began to recognise how one resident seemed to become upset as families visited others in the home. Her family lived in Canada and although they telephoned each week, the lack of contact was a source of distress for this resident. Staff wished to identify biographical details to consider significant factors appropriate to her care. This process initiated an email exchange with the family, which gave the resident much pleasure as she now had visual reminders of the contact she had (by staff printing out the emails). This led the staff to consider the use of Skype for her, the resource for which was discussed with the family.

For older people, 'ageing in place' is a broad concept, moving beyond functional issues in later life to reflect a personal meaning imbued with connections, whether these be with their neighbourhood, community, church or cultural groups (Wiles et al., 2012). In a Canadian study, community involvement for older people was positively associated with health irrespective of other issues (Zunzunegui et al., 2004). This is not to say that other limitations do not create issues for older people, with the size of housing and limitations negatively impacting on the life satisfaction of the very old (Oswald et al., 2010). However, feeling connected to the area in which they live leads to high levels of life satisfaction – the higher it is, the better their neighbourhood quality and the stronger the outdoor place attachment (Oswald et al., 2010). This suggests that for wellbeing we need to consider the relationships people have with their neighbourhood and outdoor places.

We all live in the natural world where we have access to the seasons and weather. This may be something we take for granted or a regular feature of our lives. This very much depends on our life experience, where we have grown up, the job we have done, where we have lived or the interests we have. Natural phenomena can move us emotionally; it might be the fear of a storm, the beauty of a sunset, the hope of a rainbow or the pleasure of feeling the sun on our face or the wind in our hair. Encouraging older people to access outdoor places or experience different weather is not something that forms part of the assessment process. This is surprising, given the importance of light and dark to stimulate necessary hormonal changes that enable us to sleep well and sunlight to prevent vitamin D deficiency, which can cause problems with bones (McNair, 2012).

Practice scenario: Care home

Terry spent some time as an activity coordinator at a local care home, where he would take older people for 'wheelchair walks'. These were older people for whom life had become restricted to the care home and many of them chose to go out in all weathers. When challenged by care staff, he replied that it was important for older people to feel the wind or rain on their face. When given the choice, few older people declined their opportunity to access the outdoors, irrespective of the weather, and often told him they wished they could get out more often.

The natural environment can stimulate memories, as one older woman in my research explained when she was taken out during the blackberry season and experienced the pleasure of picking blackberries as she had as a young girl (Cook and Brown Wilson, 2010). This was an example of a simple activity based on biographical knowledge the care worker had derived from the stories shared with her during care routines. Building relationships by listening to stories shared by older people is an important part of spiritual care (Mowatt, 2011). A similar story was shared by another care worker who described spiritual care as supporting an older woman to have a bird feeder at her window, which allowed her to see the birds she would have seen in her own garden and then discuss these with her family during their visits (Brown Wilson et al., 2009b). The same care worker described how being outdoors also provided a stimulus for an activity that promoted social engagement in the following case study.

Practice scenario: Care home (Brown Wilson, 2007)

One summer, Ann Marie noticed there were a number of residents in the garden, so she decided she would hold a flower arranging competition. She set up the tables and vases and made sure everyone had flowers to arrange. Everyone got into the spirit of the competition and began commenting on what each other had done. Matron was asked to judge the competition, and there was a prize for the winner. When it was finished, each arrangement was put into the resident's room for them to enjoy later. Everyone was talking about it afterwards.

This scenario demonstrates how opportunities for engaging with the outdoor world may emerge from biographical knowledge, as many older women had engaged in flower arranging as part of their domestic life. Such opportunities give people's lives meaning, which is an integral part of spirituality (Goldsmith, 2011).

There is no universal definition of spirituality and while it encompasses a religious faith, it is widely accepted that it means more than this. Depending on a person's cultural background and spiritual beliefs, contact with nature in the broadest sense is supporting the spiritual dimension of a person's life (Goldsmith, 2012). The natural world may hold the opportunity for an older person to experience the awe and magnificence of something beyond them while appreciating the immediacy of the moment. This is particularly important for people living with dementia as their condition often creates additional risks for moving freely out of doors, which minimises opportunities to interact with the natural world. This may in turn reduce confidence with the fear of becoming lost; providing opportunities for shared meaningful activities out of doors is an opportunity for a person to tap into their potential. Neil Mapes runs a company, Dementia Adventure, which supports people living with dementia and their carers to engage in outdoor activities. He outlines how people living with dementia communicate more freely and describe a sense of wellbeing during contact with the natural environment (Mapes, 2012). When we care for people with life-limiting illness, it can sometimes be easier to focus on the physical limitations of a person that may mean that person is no longer able to continue doing a particular activity.

Practice scenario: Community

Mrs Jones had a terminal condition which was reducing her mobility. Being outdoors was very important to provide her with 'peace'. The student was able to secure this woman a wheelchair, so that she could go for walks with her husband in their local park, which enabled them to continue a cherished activity within the limits of this woman's condition.

The practice scenarios in this section have demonstrated how listening to the stories people share often hold the key to significant details that may contribute to the health and wellbeing of the older people we support. Adopting a biographical approach to care provides us with information about what constitutes meaningful activity for each person. Due consideration of meaningful activity supports the spiritual, emotional and social needs of the person, while still contributing to their physical health.

Summary

Promoting 'care that matters to me' involves:

• Understanding that relationships remain an integral part of the care environment for older people, families and staff
• Recognising that older people want to feel connected to those around them but may face challenges in achieving this
• Realising that sexual expression remains an important feature in the lives of many older people, and a biographical approach to care can support nurses in addressing this important issue
• Recognising that spiritual care can be fostered by promoting connections with the natural world

Conclusion

Adopting a biographical approach enables us to consider the meaning that older people ascribe to people and places and how this has influenced the rhythm of their lives. Maintaining part of the rhythm of older people's lives that includes the seasons and outdoor environments can support people to remain connected on an emotional, social and spiritual level, while enhancing physical health and wellbeing. We have discussed the importance of intimate and sexual relationships for older people and how the natural environment provides opportunities for meaningful activities for older people, including those living with dementia and other life-limiting conditions. This chapter has provided insights into how we might ensure 'care that matters' to the older person. This will ensure we take all aspects of the older person's health and wellbeing into account, irrespective of the care context in which we work. By considering the importance of relationships in the lives of older people, we, as health care professionals, will also be able to identify the important connections for older people and how these might be maintained. Understanding how older people relate to those around them and to their wider community will enable health care professionals to anticipate the social needs older people have for emotional connection and social support.

Further reading

Dunn, K. (2011) 'Spirituality, religious practice, beliefs and values', in Reed, J., Clarke, C. and McFarlane, A. (eds), *Nursing Older People: A Textbook for Nurses*. Buckingham: Open University Press.

Gilliard, J. and Marshall, M. (eds) (2012) *Transforming the Quality of Life for People with Dementia Through Contact with the Natural World*. London: Jessica Kingsley.

Jewell, A. (ed.) *Spirituality and Personhood in Dementia*. London: Jessica Kingsley.

McAuliffe, L., Nay R. and Bauer, M. (2011) 'Sexuality and intimacy', in Reed, J., Clarke, C. and McFarlane, A. (eds), *Nursing Older People: A Textbook for Nurses*. Buckingham: Open University Press.

CHAPTER 9

Managing transitions using a biographical approach

Learning outcomes

By the end of this the chapter, the reader will be able to:

- Describe how a biographical approach might support the older person in transitions through care environments
- Consider how older people and their families might be involved in the transition process
- Critically examine the role of staff in supporting the older person to manage transitions using approaches that facilitate shared decision making
- Develop practical strategies that enable older people and their families to manage transitions while promoting their wellbeing and those around them

Introduction

This chapter draws on the underpinning theory of the developmental psychology that considers how we continue to develop across the lifespan. While later life is generally seen as a period of decline, adopting a life course perspective suggests that older people have the potential to continue to mature and develop into very old age. Approaching older people with this perspective, we begin to see through the myths and stereotypes we have explored in previous chapters to arrive at the conclusion that older people are not only able to make their own decisions but are also able to manage the outcomes of these decisions. This is not to say they will not need support to achieve this, but adopting this perspective, we are more likely to involve the older person in the decision-making process.

While developmental psychology is useful to appreciate that we develop across our lifespan from birth until death, we are also involved in a range of social processes and interactions as we adopt roles and make choices. The perspective of critical social gerontology (Minkler, 1996) challenges us to consider how social processes influence our later life. This approach questions the choices older people are able to make due to the constraints that may be placed on them by issues such as the type of work they have undertaken, and where they live. Critical gerontology highlights that when older people are unable to maintain an 'active ageing' process, it may result in further stigmatisation.

The previous chapters in this part of the book have clearly demonstrated how adopting a biographical approach enables us as practitioners to see what matters to the person. This process supports the development of shared understandings, which is an integral feature of relationship-centred care discussed in Chapter 4. A biographical approach to care enables us to understand what the health condition means to the older person and how this might impact on associations to place, people and meaningful activities. We now consider how we might use this approach to adopt strategies that involve the older person, their families and significant others in decisions that affect them.

As practitioners, we might consider the issues for older people and then present them with choices we think they should be considering. To work towards shared decision making, we need to explore different ways of involving older people beyond making them aware of the choices they have. It may be difficult for older people to navigate the health and social care system, particularly if they don't have access to the internet. Providing the right information, such as the availability of different services in the community in which the older person lives, may be a crucial factor between deciding to stay in the community or move to a supported living environment. However, there may be other transitions as older people move through different levels of care, which may require relocation. We will consider the implications of transitions through a biographical lens, drawing on information from previous chapters, and end our discussion with how to support older people as they move to the end of life.

Transitions and decision making

Older people approach their lives in different ways and it is important we understand this rather than making assumptions about their care. As we have progressed throughout this part of the book, we have considered how a biographical approach might challenge the myths and stereotypes that have developed around older age. We return to the case study of Dorothy Brown from Chapter 6 to consider how we might apply the biographical information from her assessment into decisions surrounding her discharge.

Case study: Dorothy Brown (continued)

Dorothy's home was a bungalow but being able to leave the village was dependent on her ability to drive. We saw that Dorothy's home was near the farm she grew up on and so continuing to live in this community created a range of meaningful activities through her faith network. As practitioners, we might be tempted to suggest that Dorothy should consider other living arrangements due to the need for her to drive. However, we also remember from Dorothy's biographical assessment that she did not want to move into a care home following the experience of watching her sister being cared for. Understanding the importance of living independently at home was identified as an important feature of Dorothy's biographical assessment.

In the UK, when older people come into hospital, they can expect to be actively involved in their discharge planning as equal partners (Figure 9.1). Discharge planning is a process that begins on admission, with an in-depth assessment that includes planning over an eight-day period to reduce the length of stay (DH, 2003). Staff should work within a multi-disciplinary and multi-agency team framework, encouraging active participation of older people and their carers. There are now ten steps within this process, with hospitals charged with co-ordinating this through a ward-based team that considers what is required for the potential discharge date and how best to achieve this. These steps clearly include the patient and their caregiver (DH, 2010) with penalties for delayed discharge (DH, 2009).

ACTIVITY

Planning for discharge

Return to your assessment of Dorothy from Chapter 6 and consider how this information might inform the discharge planning process as outlined in Figure 9.1. Are there any gaps between your assessment and the model? If so, what information is needed in the assessment process to capture this information?

The pressures between quick and quality discharges raise tensions for nurses, as described in a study undertaken by Michael Connolly and colleagues (2008). When asked about discharge planning, nurses expressed concern at their lack of time to assess patients, the overly complex paperwork and the difficulties in communication within the hospital and with external services, which led to a sense of depersonalisation of care (Connolly et al., 2009). Adopting a biographical approach to assessment, as we did in Chapter 6, has the potential to address some of these issues, if we use our assessment to consider what matters to the older person, both in their immediate care and in their plans for discharge.

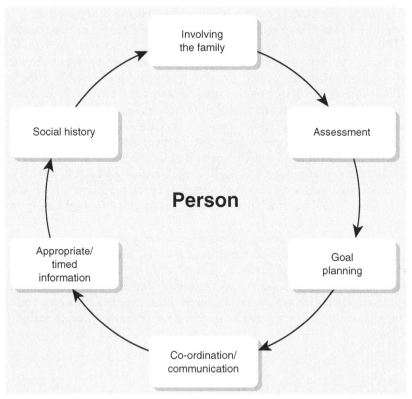

Figure 9.1 Creating a person-centred discharge process

Case study: Dorothy Brown (continued)

Returning to Dorothy, we can see from our assessment that for such an independent person, she would be aiming for a relatively quick discharge, but as she also lives alone, she would benefit from a period of intermediate care to ensure she regains sufficient mobility and independence to be safe at home. For Dorothy, it would be important to consider the social support system she had in place as she had limited family support and this would impact on the amount of time she would require in transitional care. Dorothy's discharge planning would include discussions with Dorothy as to the location of appropriate intermediate care beds and a discussion of her future needs, which the re-ablement team could then support. For Dorothy, it was important she was close to her community, so she felt there was not too much strain placed on those who were supporting her.

Increasing intermediate care beds for older people remains a key aspiration for government policy in the UK to reduce the need for older people to remain in hospital (Philp, 2006). Older people require more time for rehabilitation and acute care is not necessarily the appropriate environment as older people are more at risk of hospital-acquired infections, which increases their length of stay. Dorothy was discharged to a care home that provided intermediate care. However, the cost of care in an environment in which she felt comfortable raised concerns for Dorothy. In Chapter 7, we saw the importance of place and the communities in which older people live. A European study found that participants living in more accessible homes, who perceive their home as meaningful, are more independent in daily activities and have a better sense of wellbeing (Oswald et al., 2007). This suggests that for an effective discharge we might need to develop a better understanding of the lives older people live, which occurs when we adopt a biographical approach to assessment.

In our case study of Dorothy, there were never concerns that she would be discharged anywhere but the community; however, for many older people with co-morbidities, the discharge planning process may be more complex. Adopting a biographical approach to assessment, as we did for Dorothy, supports older people in making known what is important to them in the longer term at the time of admission, which then contributes to the discharge-planning process, without making this a separate task.

Transitions in care delivery

Working across disciplines is very important when we consider how we might support older people to remain independent. Ensuring appropriate referrals to occupational therapy, physiotherapy and social work are integral if we are to support older people in living meaningful lives as they manage their health and illness. An underused resource in this area is assistive technology that may enable older people with life-limiting illness, including dementia, to remain living independently within the community. Smart technology has been developed to support older people to 'age in place', providing technological solutions that will facilitate older people to live at home. Roger Orpwood and colleagues in Bath, for example, are developing useful devices to facilitate the safe use of water taps, gas cookers and lamps, and are including people with dementia in the design process (Orpwood et al., 2004). Applying technology to everyday items used in a home environment can overcome difficulties for people living with dementia and allay caregiver concern. It is also possible to use sensor technology within homes and GPS technology outside the home to monitor a person's movements. While ethical concerns have been raised about this, there is some evidence that these technologies provide support for caregivers in the community and people with dementia find them acceptable (Robinson et al., 2006). However, there are also more simple technological aids, as Dorothy's continuing case study demonstrates.

Case study: Dorothy Brown (continued)

On asking Dorothy about safety conditions in her home it became clear that she had undertaken a range of house alterations as she had aged. This has included fitting a shower instead of a bath and asking Age UK to support her with modifications such as grab rails and more accessible stairs both inside and outside her bungalow. In her assessment, we also found that Dorothy had purchased a personal alarm system, which she was able to use when she fell prior to her surgery. These are simple technologies that Dorothy chose to manage the environment in which she lived, enabling her to maintain an independent lifestyle.

Sheila Peace and colleagues (2011) describe this ongoing process of assessment, calibration and adjustment as options recognition, where older people consider how they are able to maintain their self-identity in relation to the difficulties they face in their environment, at both the personal and community level. These adaptations are potentially the difference between older people living independently or needing to move into residential care. While such technology concentrates on supporting people to physically stay at home, we also need to consider other aspects of their lives. Therefore, home modification and relocation should not be prescribed but need to be negotiated with older adults to take into account their personal preferences (Oswald et al., 2007).

An essential part of the discharge-planning process mentioned earlier is assessing the needs of caregivers. In a systematic review of family caregiving relationships involving people with dementia, Quinn and colleagues (2009) conclude that caregiving can have an impact on the quality of the relationship between the caregiver and the care recipient with pre-caregiving and current relationship quality influencing the caregiver's wellbeing. Much of the literature about caregiving focuses on emotional strain and burden, with limited studies considering the positive nature of this relationship (Nolan et al., 1996). Philip Clissett (2007) found that caregiving often resulted in spending more time together and this could be viewed both negatively and positively. Seeing caregiving as a disruption to the previous relationship tended to have more negative consequences but could be reversed with the support of a professional caregiver (Clissett, 2007). Carbonneau and colleagues (2010) have undertaken a further review of the literature and describe a positive model of relationships in caregiving as being dependent on the quality of day-to-day caregiver and care receiver relationship. The care recipient's need for help with the activities of daily living and the level of behavioural problems are important factors that influence the caregiver's perceptions of relationship quality (Quinn et al., 2009). Underpinned by the concept of the caregiver's self-efficacy, Carbonneau et al.'s (2010) model suggests that positive aspects of the caregiving relationship are derived from the meaning the caregiver ascribes to their role in daily life activities, feeling able to engage in activities that provide enrichment, which contribute to the caregiver's feeling of accomplishment. The components of this model are inter-dependent and reinforce the caregiver's wellbeing, which supports ongoing involvement in caregiving.

Providing caregiver support within the community is integral to enabling older people to remain in their own homes. This might take the form of practical solutions such as respite care or support with the activities of living using domiciliary care agencies. This support is not without its problems, as there may be issues to consider such as the timing for home care support and how workload is allocated for these workers. This service, as with respite provided by social care, is means-tested in the UK and so many people will need to pay towards this care. Family caregivers often raise concern as to how supportive (or not) such services may be, at times preferring to have no service at all due to the disruption caused in daily routines, not knowing who may be coming to deliver care or the standard of care being provided. While this may vary between regions and according to the home care agency or respite environment, it suggests that support for caregivers might not be as consistent or supportive as is needed. The absence of caregivers or their inability to continue with providing care is a key risk factor for moving older people, particularly those with dementia, into residential environments.

Transitions between places

There will be some older people for whom returning to their home in the community will not be possible. When older people are considering changes to their lives, we shouldn't forget the emotive issues that may emerge with this as a person's home will be imbued with symbolic meaning and emotional attachments (Andrews et al., 2007). Relocating from a person's own home to a care home can be very traumatic as a familiar place with treasured memories is lost. Older people describe a 'good life' in old age, consisting of social relationships with family, friends and neighbours, a sense of belonging within a wider community and leisure pursuits or activities that provide pleasure and stimulation (Godfrey et al., 2004). Knowing what 'a good life' means to the older person can provide opportunities for supporting them in decision making that moves beyond information giving. This is particularly important when supporting people with dementia, as decisions may be considered by both family and professionals as beyond them, as demonstrated in the following practice scenario.

Practice scenario: Community

Mary had dementia and lived in sheltered accommodation. She explained that she used to have lots of friends but since having memory problems, she hadn't been

(Continued)

(Continued)

out much and at times felt very lonely in her flat. This meant that often her brother would come when she was being seen by health care professionals, who frequently spoke directly to Mary's brother. Using a biographical approach, the student found that Mary was feeling isolated and that her view did not count. She was encouraged to express her own views and a local day centre was found to support Mary in making friends in the locality. This demonstrates that we must not assume that all people with dementia are not able to understand our conversation or be involved in the decision-making process.

We know that family members of people with dementia are often influenced by safety concerns (Kelsey et al., 2010) whereas the person with dementia may wish to continue to take certain risks to maintain meaningful activity in their lives. Thein and colleagues (2011) interviewed people with dementia before and after a move and found the lack of active involvement in the process can lead to the older person feeling left out and having a sense of loss of control over their own lives. Conversely, moving to residential care can be a positive move for a person with dementia when involved in decision making when having opportunities for a pre-move visit (Thein et al., 2011). A number of studies have been able to demonstrate that people with dementia are capable of being involved in the decision-making process (Thein et al., 2011). However, when this is not possible it may fall to the nurse to facilitate an assessment of capacity for a person with dementia (Mental Capacity Act, 2008). Further support in decision making is also possible through an independent mental capacity advocate (IMCA). Undertaking best interest meetings that involve all stakeholders is essential to ensure an appropriate decision-making process for people with dementia who are no longer able to make such decisions have been realised for themselves.

It is perhaps not surprising that older people who feel they have no choice over relocation will not respond as well as those for whom relocation has been an active choice and is well planned (Chao et al., 2008). This is also true for family caregivers involved in the move, with more positive experience being described when families felt they were able to work in partnership with staff to positively influence the transition for their relative (Davies and Nolan, 2004). In their in-depth qualitative study, Rossen and Knafl (2003) found that for older people, being able to maintain meaningful routines helped the transition process. Feeling competent in the new environment and developing new relationships also supports integration into the social network of the new environment (Rossen and Knafl, 2003). This underpins the importance of staff supporting the development of social networks between older people within communal living environments, which we discussed in Chapter 8.

ACTIVITY

Return to the person who was involved in a move from your activities in Chapters 7 and 8

- What were the key concerns expressed by the older person in the transition process?
- What biographical information was helpful in that transition process?
- Was this information recorded and/or shared between organisations?
- What might improve this process?

A number of housing options are available for older people in the UK, USA and Australia that involve living in supported communities where all levels of care are provided. However, within these communities, people still need to move within the community when different levels of care are required (Cheek et al., 2007). Although this may seem to be only a small transition, it has been found to disrupt social networks that have been developed when health care needs mean a change in the living environment is required (Shippee, 2009). Such changes are often precipitated by a gradual decline in abilities but may also be influenced by the opportunity to move when a place becomes available in the co-located residential facility (Cheek et al., 2007). Transitions may also be enforced such as when facilities close. In a Canadian study, Coughlan and Ward (2007) found that even when the move was to an improved environment, it disrupted relationships with both staff and other residents, which were central to their perception of the quality of care they received (Coughlan and Ward, 2007). Jan Reed and colleagues (2003) undertook a study that considered transition between levels of care in the UK and suggest that residents' involvement in decisions to move between care homes (due to closure or when care needs escalate) can be considered along a continuum between active involvement to passive acquiescence (Reed et al., 2003). This may be different for people living with dementia, when the decision to move into a specialist care environment may be taken by staff and family members (Kelsey et al., 2010). In a large study involving assisted living facilities and care homes in the USA, Sheryl Zimmerman and colleagues (2005) suggest that the most significant areas that influence quality of life for people with dementia include having staff with specialist knowledge and consistent staff assignment where people are encouraged to participate in meaningful activity (Zimmerman et al., 2005).

The transition to higher levels of care makes the assumption that older people's condition will not improve, but simply continue to decline. This has been challenged in an assisted living facility in the USA, where Marilyn Rantz and colleagues have used a range of sensor technology to identify early onset of illness by alerting the nurse co-ordinator to changes in activity patterns and vital signs (Alexander et al., 2011). Conditions such as urinary tract infections and chest infections might be detected earlier and treated before they reach a severity that may result in hospital admission (Rantz et al., 2011). This means that by using this technology, skilled nursing care can be brought into the facility when the older person requires this and then withdrawn as the person's condition improves (Rantz et al., 2010). This is aimed at ensuring any period of health decline might be less acute and so cause less functional disability as the person ages and so they are able to 'age in place' (Rantz et al., 2005).

The literature we have considered so far suggests there is a role for staff and the wider organisation within the transition process. From a literature review undertaken by the National Care Homes Research and Development Forum (2007), *My Home Life*, a national initiative (www.myhomelife.org), has suggested 'top tips' for supporting older people and families when involved in transitions to care homes. These include having trial visits, bringing in items that hold treasured memories, promoting social contacts within the home and involving the older person in the decision-making process. This brings us back to the importance of a biographical assessment when moving between care environments and identifying how important information might be shared between staff across organisational boundaries.

Transition towards the end of life

Palliative care is an approach that improves the quality of life for older people when faced with life-threatening illness through the prevention and relief of suffering adopting a team approach (WHO, 2003). Palliative care interventions generally include the assessment and management of physical, psychological and spiritual symptoms and advance care planning (Hall et al., 2011).

As practitioners, we need to be considering our role in supporting older people to communicate their wishes for care as they move towards the end of life. Advance care planning (ACP) using documentation such as the preferred priorities of care (PPC) developed in the UK as part of the end of life care strategy (DH, 2008) may support us in this process. PPC is a patient-held document that has been designed to support multi-disciplinary care decisions as a person's condition deteriorates, reducing the need for hospitalisation or unwanted interventions at the end of life.

Practice scenario: Community

Mrs Jenkins had been a keen gardener and cherished her garden of 30 years. She was coming to the last stages of life in spring time which was her favorite time in the gardon. She wanted to stay at home but was concerned about her husband being able to manage her personal care. She wished to continue to do this herself. The staff put in place equipment to promote Mrs Jenkins' independence at home to prevent her becoming bed bound. This action enabled Mrs Jenkins to remain at home, supported by her husband and able to enjoy the garden she loved.

To support us in considering the transition towards the end of life, we need to ask the surprise question: Would you be surprised if this person were to die sometime in the near future? If the answer is no, we should ask about preferred priorities of care, using a hypothetical question: If something was to happen to you and you were unable to contribute towards making a decision about ..., what would you like to happen? It may be important to involve families in discussions about 'What might happen if ...', to support them in coming to terms with their relative's end of life and the decisions that the older person may have communicated previously. In a systematic review of multi-component palliative care interventions within care homes, Hall et al. (2011) found that developing palliative care expertise in care homes, referring on to specialist services and moving residents with end-stage dementia to special units in the care home had the most promising results.

When given the choice, many older people would not choose to die in hospital but in an environment surrounded by people known to them. To this end, hospitals in the UK have now instituted rapid discharge schemes facilitating this choice. The implementation of the Gold Standards Framework (GSF) and the use of the Liverpool Care Pathway (LCP) within the community are deemed to positively support the choice of many older people who may wish to die in their home. The GSF is aimed at promoting a greater awareness of the trajectory leading to the end of life, usually in the last three to six months of life, and the LCP then provides a framework upon which to manage the last few days of life.

The GSF has also been developed for care homes where the focus is on promoting positive relationships with care professionals in the wider community, as well as ensuring staff have the skills and expertise to support people at the end of life. There is some evidence to suggest that this programme increases advance care planning and reduces crisis admission to hospital at the end of life (Badger et al., 2009). Knowledge and skills are important when considering the ability to involve older people and families in the decision-making process about preferred priorities of care, to recognise when people are moving along the trajectory to imminent death, the ability to manage symptom control and being able to support families (Parker and Froggatt, 2011). A relationship-centred approach may facilitate good end-of-life care as it takes into account the needs of all within the relationship, the older person, the family and staff.

Identifying when a person is reaching the end of their life remains problematic for many older people who may have a range of co-morbid conditions irrespective of the context of their death. Although many care home managers understand the importance of discussions around preferred priorities of care, the completion of advance care planning documentation in care homes remains sporadic, which has been attributed to a lack of confidence and knowledge with respect to end-of-life care, ACP and related communication with residents and relatives (Froggatt et al., 2009). Effective end-of-life care in care homes is also influenced by external factors such as professional support by district nurses and general practitioners (GPs) in the wider community, access to resources such as syringe drivers and end-of-life training, which influences the ability of the home to support older people at the end of life (Seymour et al., 2011).

For those who wish to die at home but have no family caregiver support, professional services remain concerned with being able to provide the level of care required in terminal phases (Rolls et al., 2011). Even when family caregivers are available, they require support in the practical aspects of caring for a dying relative, including information about the disease process (Funk et al., 2010). Although there is some evidence to suggest that supporting family caregivers at the end of life requires a personalised approach (Funk et al., 2010), there is limited evidence on appropriate interventions that will improve caregiver outcomes (Stajduhar et al., 2010). Supporting people with dementia at the end of life also remains problematic with limited research in this area on which to base decisions. People with dementia tend to have a poorer experience of dying due to the unique circumstances created by the dementia not being taken into account (Lawrence et al., 2011). This is further complicated by a limited recognition as to when people stop living with dementia and begin dying with dementia, meaning that many people with dementia may end up being transferred to hospital at the end of their life (Goodman et al., 2010). Good end-of-life care is possible when care plans are developed with the family and there is co-ordination between services to ensure these are followed, including the avoidance of transfer to acute hospitals (Lawrence et al., 2011).

Suppporting decision making at the end of life

Return to the previous activity and check it for any information that would provide support for introducing a discussion about advance care planning. You might consider:

- Would this person be happy to go to hospital, should they fall ill?
- If this person got a very bad infection, would they want it treated?
- Where would this person choose to die?
- How might you involve the family in this decision-making process?

ACTIVITY

Although the evidence for end-of-life care is not robust, we can consider how a biographical approach might support us in allowing the older person to raise issues that may be on their mind. This is particularly important for older people who may live alone, such as with our case study of Dorothy Brown. We heard from her biographical assessment in Chapter 6 that Dorothy is very independent and wishes to remain living in her own home; we also know that she would not wish to die in a care home as her sister did. This may lead us to a suggestion that Dorothy might like to consider completing a PPC document, which could then go with her at the time of subsequent admissions to hospital should she not be able to contribute to the discussions about her care. This is the starting point for all older people to involve them in the decision-making process.

One of the limitations of the PPC documentation is that it assumes the older person is able to communicate verbally. This may not be possible with all older people, particularly those who live with dementia. This is when a biographical approach can be very helpful in that it supports professional staff in taking into account the person's background and how they approached their life prior to the onset of dementia. Involving families and significant others provides a more effective approach in decision making, particularly in late stage dementia (Caron et al., 2005), and these meetings or conversations can be recorded as best interest conversations.

Assessment and care planning moving towards the end of life needs to consider the physical, social, emotional and spiritual needs of the older person. Adopting a biographical assessment in this respect can be very helpful. Listening to stories of how other family members have died and the feelings this has left the older person with, may provide opportunities to explore what a 'good death' might mean for this person. A biographical assessment may also provide insights into how to approach issues of physical symptoms such as pain relief as well as personal knowledge that will support nutrition and hydration. Ensuring GPs are involved in the decision-making process and out-of-hours services are advised can often prevent unnecessary hospital admissions at the end of life, so the older person is enabled to die in an environment where they know the staff. When this does not happen, it can be distressing for both the older person and the staff (Seymour et al., 2011).

> Good end of life care doesn't end at the point of death: one care home involves other residents in celebrating the lives of people who have died by having a remembrance book and memorial garden. Staff and residents also need to feel comfortable in expressing their feelings when someone dies. (www.myhomelife.org)

Lawrence and colleagues (2011) suggested that meeting physical care needs in a way that moved beyond task-focused care supported effective palliative care for people with dementia. Care delivery at the end of life needs to be individualised and delivered with compassion, demonstrating that the staff know what matters to both the dying person and their family (Lawrence et al., 2011). This underpins the importance of a biographical assessment. However, when caring for the dying, staff may also experience negative emotions and require support. Adopting a relationship-centred approach (see Chapter 4) that recognises the needs of the staff, alongside the needs of the older person and their family, may promote a compassionate approach to end of life care.

Summary

Promoting 'care that involves us all' involves:

- Developing biographical knowledge, which develops shared understandings between older people, families and staff, contributing towards decision making
- Transitions for older people, which may involve physical relocation or different levels of care in one environment
- Supporting older people towards the end of life, which involves anticipating care needs and involving older people, families and other professionals in decision making

Conclusion

Many older people will experience transitions across the health and social care system. We can see from our discussions that not all of these transitions will be due to increasing disability, with some transitions providing opportunities for increased independence or reducing disability. Working with families and across organisational boundaries will support older people as they manage transition. Transitions may be between institutions, between care providers or between levels of care, involving more specialist practitioners such as when supporting people with dementia or managing the transition to end of life. Adopting a biographical approach to assessment facilitates the involvement of the older person in the decision-making process, as it provides opportunities to discuss goals, aspirations and concerns. This promotes shared understandings contributing to effective decision making, which will impact on the transitional process.

Further reading

Clarke, A. and Smith, P. (2011) 'Dying', in Reed, J., Clarke, C. and McFarlane, A. (eds), *Nursing Older People: A Textbook for Nurses*. Buckingham: Open University Press.
Parker, D. and Froggatt, K. (2011) 'Palliative care with older people', in Tolson, D., Booth, J. and Schofield, I. (eds), *Evidence Informed Nursing with Older People*. Oxford: Wiley Blackwell.

Other resources

Department of Health *Prevention Package for Older People*. Downloadable resources. London: Department of Health. Available at: www.dh.gov.uk/
Preferred priorities of care. Available at: www.endoflifecareforadults.nhs.uk/tools/core-tools/preferredprioritiesforcare
The Route to Success care programme. Available at: www.endoflifecare.nhs.uk/routes_to_success/

CHAPTER 10

Valuing the contribution of older people, families and staff: implications for practice

Learning outcomes

After reading this chapter, the student will be able to:

- Examine how leadership, motivation of staff and teamwork might support them in adopting person-centred or relationship-centred approaches to care
- Describe how the contributions made by older people and families might be facilitated supporting more participatory approaches to care
- Critically examine how a biographical assessment might influence outcomes of care
- Consider how the experience of the older person might be assessed within established quality mechanisms

Introduction

When supporting older people, we may subconsciously revert to seeing older people through the lens of chronological age rather than considering their full potential to lead a fulfilling and interesting life. In adopting a biographical approach, we challenge the stereotyping of chronological age and see what is possible even at advanced ages. The judgements we make as practitioners will have an impact on how we involve the older person in the decision-making process and the opportunities they will have to regain functional ability and so lead a life they choose.

In Chapter 1, we considered the different models of care in the literature according to the extent to which each approach actively encouraged the participation of the older person, family caregiver and staff. This has helped us differentiate between the different models of individualised, person and relationship centred care in the literature and demonstrated that there might not be a 'one size fits all' approach. Underpinning this were my observations of staff adopting different approaches at different times in their care; mealtimes were an example where staff who might usually adopt a relationship-centred approach, tended towards an individualised task-centred approach (Brown Wilson, 2007). When I asked staff why this was, they spoke about the importance of ensuring everyone had a hot meal and were supported to eat this wherever they chose, which might have been in the communal dining room, or their own room. Staff felt an individualised task-centred approach was the best way of ensuring everyone's nutritional needs were met. However, I also observed the same staff move back to a relationship-centred approach at other times, where they felt they had more flexibility. This was consistent across my research as I also observed staff who generally adopted an individualised task-centred approach alter their practice to adopt a person-centred or relationship-centred approach. In concluding Chapter 1, we inferred that involving the older person, family and staff in the decision-making process would increase their participation and so improve care outcomes.

This led us to explore the three approaches to care (individualised, person and relationship centred) in Chapters 2–4. Within each of these chapters, we reviewed evidence from care homes, the community and acute care contexts in how each of these approaches impacted on the care of older people and the contribution they and their families were able to make to their care. As we progressed through these chapters, we were able to see the improved experience for older people, families and staff as everyone became more involved in both the care routines and the wider community. We concluded in Chapter 5 that each of these approaches led to a different level of experience for older people, families and staff, with the most positive experiences occuring where 'care involved us all' through a relationship-centred approach (Figure 5.1).

Part 2 began with an introduction to how myths and stereotypes might influence our practice and the importance of understanding our personal values when supporting older people. This part focused on how we might implement the approaches from Part 1 to improve specific aspects of care for the older person. Chapter 6 presented a case study of an older person who required support with her mobility and we examined how a biographical approach to her care could improve the patient journey. Building on the biographical approach, we then investigated how people connect with their environment (Chapter 7) and those around them (Chapter 8). Within each of these chapters, we considered both physical and psychosocial needs and how adopting a biographical approach to care promoted individualised, person-centred or relationship-centred care. We concluded this part (Chapter 9) by discussing how we might support older people and their families through transitions of care between care environments, between levels of care and towards the end of life.

I have argued throughout this book that by valuing the contribution of older people, families and staff, we are more likely to adopt a person-centred or relationship-centred approach. In this chapter, we bring together the key messages within this book and determine how we might positively influence the care of older people. This includes how we encourage and value the contribution of older people and their families, how we work together in teams and how we provide leadership in the care environment in which we work. Improving care for older people starts with one person and making changes in practice is similar. We might want to start at the individualised task-centred approach and then steer staff towards more person-centred strategies as they recognise the benefits this holds for the care of older people. Adopting this pragmatic approach to care might facilitate the adoption of small changes in everyday practice that may then have a positive impact on the care of older people and the experience of families. Once staff recognise how a biographical approach promotes involvement of the older person and their family, these staff members are more likely to develop shared understandings that support a relationship-centred approach. If we ask staff to work differently, we also need to be able to capture this work in established quality cycles to prevent it from becoming invisible work. Considering how we capture the experience of older people and their families is one way to address this issue and one we will be exploring in this final chapter.

Using leadership, motivation and teamwork to influence the care of older people

In the first part of this book, we considered the different attributes of leadership, staff motivation and teamwork that might promote an individualised task-centred, person- or relationship-centred approach to care. Leadership that was driven from the front of the organisation tended to foster an individualised task-centred approach across the organisation (Chapter 2). This style of leadership was more rule-based and as such encouraged staff to make sure all the tasks of care were achieved. Such rule-based leadership was in direct contrast to leadership that led by example (Chapter 4). Leading by example enabled staff to adopt a more flexible approach, taking into account shared understandings promoting opportunities for negotiation and compromise. We established that leadership is more than management and that leadership can happen at all levels within an organisation. Even with a rules-based approach to leadership from management, it is possible to implement person-centred strategies in an individual's approach to practice. The challenge here is to demonstrate to management how person-centred strategies might improve the experience of the older person. Capturing this information will be something we return to later in this chapter.

Motivation of staff is influential in the approaches to care they adopt. McCormack and McCance (2006) describe one of the attributes of a nurse as dedication to providing care that is best for the person. Staff in my research described the belief that adopting a task-centred approach to care was providing the best care for the person, which supported an individualised task-centred approach. The motivation staff described in adopting a person-centred approach to care was 'to do unto others' (Chapter 3). This meant that staff considered care delivery from the perspective of the older person and made every effort to implement care that mattered to that person, as this was how they would like care delivered if they or someone close to them were in that position. Staff adopting a person-centred approach also described coming into the care industry to 'make a difference' to people's lives. Developing a relationship-centred approach required staff with a motivation of 'doing what was right for all of us' (Chapter 4). The key difference in adopting a relationship-centred approach was the equal recognition of the perspectives of the older person, the families and staff in the situation. A relationship-centred approach recognised how situations might change and that it was important to involve everyone in the decision-making process. Understanding the motivation of staff is one way that we might consider how to move between approaches. For example, in Chapter 5 we discussed how redefining care as 'care that mattered' from the perspective of the older person was one way of encouraging staff to adopt a person-centred approach.

Teamwork is vital if we are to provide a co-ordinated approach to caring for older people and is necessary irrespective of what approach we adopt. Having a critical mass of staff that subscribe to the same motivation will influence the dominant approach adopted within a care environment. Moving a care environment from one approach to another is often outside the ability of student practitioners. However, it is possible to influence team members by role modelling good practice (Box 10.1). To promote person-centred care, students could undertake a biographical assessment of one older person in the care environment and share the results of this with other team members, thus involving the wider team in the decision-making process.

Box 10.1   What we can do as students to role model good practice

- Individualise care by getting to know the patient – offering choice/likes/dislikes
- Undertake a biographical assessment that takes into account the older person's life experience, approach to their health/condition and their aspirations
- Put significant details from biographical assessment into place, i.e. use in care planning and communicate to rest of team (including multi-disciplinary team)
- Involve families in developing the biographical assessment by encouraging them to communicate their needs and concerns – develop shared understandings by sensitive communication between three parties
- Engage in negotiation and compromise between the three parties to ensure all needs are taken into account

Undertaking a biographical assessment provides details about the older person and family that enable all perspectives to be taken into account. As practitioners, we need to be able to articulate how a biographical assessment benefits the older person and how this information informs care. Demonstrating how this information also improves the organisation of care will provide a compelling argument that will be difficult for staff to ignore.

A key tenet of the relationship-centred approach in Chapter 4 was the ability to negotiate and compromise, which is a skill we need to consider as we move from student to practitioner. A starting point in adopting a relationship-centred approach to care would be an individual practitioner entering into negotiation and seeking compromises with other staff to improve the care of the older person. However, this approach is more likely to require a critical mass of staff who are willing to enter into negotiation and be prepared to compromise (Chapter 4). Understanding staff motivation is a useful starting point that may help us frame our negotiation in terms of what 'makes sense' to an individual practitioner (Corazzini et al., 2004). For example, if the motivation of staff is 'to do a good job' then the benefits to the organisation of care might be highlighted first. This would be in contrast to the motivation of 'making a difference' where the benefit to the older person might be at the forefront of the negotiation (Box 10.2).

Box 10.2   Role modelling good practice as a practitioner

- Demonstrate leadership in adopting a biographical approach and making associated changes in the environment
- Negotiate the above with the team for one person
- Consider the motivation of staff and pitch the importance of biographical assessment in terms of this motivation, i.e. to do a good job = to make a difference in the lives of older people and their families
- Promote wider teamwork that engages with the biographical assessment of other older people
- Support staff in developing negotiation skills
- Support flexible working practices that enable care to meet the needs of older people, families and staff

We have considered the importance of leadership, motivation and teamwork. These are important elements of the structure in our quality model (Chapter 5). It can be difficult to map these issues to a particular patient outcome. There is limited research on the attributes of leaders and teams that promote a person-centred or relationship-centred approach. Defining these attributes would be a first step towards developing appropriate tools, to demonstrate how leaders and teams may directly influence the patient experience of 'care that matters to me' and 'care that involves us all'.

Facilitating the contributions of older people and families

Patient stories and narratives are becoming increasingly recognised as important ways in which we understand the perspective of the older person as 'patient', 'client' or 'service user'. I have outlined how the stories older people and families share are often an unrecognised mechanism by which they contribute to their care (Chapter 2). Adopting a more person-centred approach to care recognises the value of these stories, and we saw examples of how staff used these stories to develop the care plan incorporating significant details into the care of the older person (Chapter 3). This was on the whole an organic process although there have been specific tools applied to extracting relevant information from patient stories (McCormack and McCance, 2010). I have not advocated a specific way of using patient stories but highlighted some simple but useful strategies (Chapter 6). Older people and families who shared stories with staff communicated their desire to develop more personal relationships, and a person-centred approach is more likely to be adopted when staff recognise and value these stories.

A biographical assessment (Chapter 6) demonstrates how we might value the stories shared by older people and families through incorporating this information into care planning. This facilitates involvement in the care process as significant details are shared and recorded in the care plan. A biographical approach also generates information about shared routines with family members which may include special outings that enable older people and families to maintain their connections (Chapter 8). Involving the family in a biographical assessment enables the contributions from the family to be valued. If the family wish to remain involved in direct care giving, meeting the needs of their loved one, then this promotes a person-centred approach. However, older people and families also make contributions beyond their immediate care to support others in the care environment (Chapter 4), contributing to the wider community of care. Inviting families to contribute to routines supports the development of shared understandings. We saw how this might include asking families their perspective during ward rounds or involving them in communal routines in care homes. This enables families to feel part of the community within the care environment and facilitates a relationship-centred approach as they consider how they might support the needs of others in the wider community. However, there is limited guidance on how this might be captured in everyday practice. Paperwork is often medically dominated, or in social care focused on the person. There is rarely the opportunity for the needs of families or aspirations of families to be recorded. This means that often the contribution of families may go unnoticed or be misunderstood. Adopting a relationship-centred approach is a starting point in recognising the contribution of families and appropriately involving them in care decisions.

Creating a sense of community (Brown Wilson, 2009) begins with the recognition that everyone within the community has a contribution to make. It can sometimes be difficult to see this when we are in busy environments confronted by the complex needs of frail older people. A biographical assessment enables us to consider the person, their interests, their family and wider relationships (Chapter 8). Older people may wish to be actively involved in the community and staff have a responsibility to consider how older people might be supported to make a valued contribution. Recognising the potential of older people is the first step in staff facilitating their contribution to the wider community and so promoting a relationship-centred approach. I have advocated that this contribution promotes the wellbeing of the older person (Chapter 8), which has been suggested as an outcome for person-centred care (McCormack and McCance, 2010). However, there has been little written that considers how the contribution of older people and their families might be captured within the quality process. This may be due to the difficulty of measuring this concept or linking it with current outcome measures.

Measuring appropriate outcomes

We discussed how it can be difficult to associate the process of nursing care with specific outcomes as nurses are often part of a multi-disciplinary team (Chapter 5). Nurse-sensitive outcomes have been developed internationally but remain focused on the tasks that lead to these outcomes (Nakrem et al., 2009). It is not always clear how the actions of the nurse influence specific outcomes beyond the task, which remains problematic when we consider patient experience as a relevant outcome. We have argued, for example, that satisfaction with care describes the experience of older people who may receive an individualised task-centred approach where their choices and preferences are met but they might not be involved in their care beyond advising staff and staff then responding accordingly (Chapter 5).

Health care is now looking at how businesses gather customer satisfaction data using similar strategies to gain more in-depth information about the patient experience. Using technology, health care organisations can produce their own questionnaires to demonstrate how their service is responding to local needs and government priorities. Technology also enables large amounts of data to be collected and then analysed according to patient group. This is particularly useful when assessing the needs of frail older people or people with specific conditions such as dementia. Technology allows people to feed back at the point of experience, ensuring a level of responsiveness to patient needs not previously possible. This can be achieved via a tablet, through apps, using touch screens or online. While older people may experience difficulty when using technology (Tolson and Brown Wilson, 2011), in research conducted by Coventry University, 63% of people over 65 were comfortable with touch screens, but this figure plummeted to 12% for online satisfaction surveys (Thompson and Sheth, 2008).

Many questionnaires may ask a global question such as: How satisfied are you with your care? While such broad questions may provide a valid measure, it is difficult to assess how this outcome is linked to a specific process. Identifying who is involved in someone's care and examining their approach might make these data more meaningful, but it is again problematic in areas where there are large teams working together. Equally, there are some older people who may not have high expectations of the care they receive.

Different environments may measure satisfaction in different ways. For example, some areas in the NHS have developed care cards that enable patients to identify which of eight different areas matter to them in their care (self-confidence; respect; reassurance; effectiveness; safety; comfort; understanding; honesty). The care cards support staff to initiate conversations with older people to find out what matters to them. This enables staff to address concerns patients may have in real time, improving the patient experience. This is a person-centred process that is potentially measurable while still capturing the different issues that matter to an older person.

In Chapter 6, we explored how a biographical assessment might be used to find out care priorities from the person's perspective. If we intend measuring the outcome of 'care that matters to me', we need to consider what aspects of the biographical assessment process we can define and measure. Using the activities of living as a conversation guide in our assessment enabled us to ascertain what mattered to Dorothy Brown and use this in the care-planning process. Auditing the assessment documentation for biographical details and then following how these were addressed within patient records may be one way of measuring the outcome of care that 'matters to me' and associating this with the assessment process. This infers we might need to consider how we document biographical details as a legitimate source of information within patient records. This goes beyond a social history to being able to follow how details have been included in the care plan and then evaluated. To achieve this, we need to ask whether the organisation is investing in the structure of leadership and teamwork.

The difficulties of associating structure with specific outcomes were discussed earlier in this chapter. If we are going to audit how staff undertake a biographical assessment, it would also be useful to consider if there is appropriate leadership in place and to assess how management supports these leaders. We might also wish to consider if there is a critical mass of staff enabling relationships to develop and biographical information to be enacted within care routines. Staff recruitment and retention is also something that will impact on teamwork and the philosophy of a care environment. One question that has been put to me is whether we should be using motivation as a mechanism for recruiting staff. If we are aiming for an ethos of person/relationship-centred approaches to care, then the next logical step would be to recruit staff with the appropriate motivation.

In moving from a person-centred approach that supports the outcome of 'care that matters to me' to a relationship-centred approach that supports the outcome of 'care that involves us all', we need to consider how we might capture (and measure) the contribution of older people and families. This remains problematic as many older people and families might contribute in different ways. When considering how to capture such contributions, it might be useful to reflect whether older people and families are encouraged to make contributions and if this is indeed something that interests them. This might take the form of a series of questions that reflect the experience of older people and their families as a consequence of a person-centred (Chapter 3) or relationship-centred (Chapter 4) processes (Table 10.1). Promoting Relationships in Care Environments (PRiCE) (Chapter 5) suggests it is possible to adopt more than one approach to care and that staff may move between approaches. It would be preferable for staff to adopt the approach that provided the best experience for older people, families and staff but there is also the recognition that this might not be possible at all times. A simple questionnaire, such as the one suggested in Table 10.1, would enable the care environment to identify the experience of the older person and their family and then support staff in moving towards a more relationship-centred approach that involved everyone in the relationship. In Table 10.1, I have included a column that allows the person to say if something is not of interest. For example, not all older people wish to be involved in their care and so by saying they do not wish to be involved preventing a false negative response to this question.

Other tools for capturing the experience of older people, families and staff have been developed for long-term care. Using the Senses Framework (see Chapter 1), Faulkner et al. (2006) developed the CARE Profiles, which comprise three structured questionnaires for older people, families and staff. These Profiles were developed with all stakeholders in care homes, and each questionnaire reflects elements from each Sense (security, significance, continuity, belonging, purpose, achievement) from the perspective of older people, families and staff. These questionnaires are quite long and generally expect people to be able to recall their experience of the past month or week, which may be difficult for older people, particularly those with dementia. A conversational approach to questionnaires may promote the involvement of people with mild to moderate dementia, but observational methods are generally needed for people with advanced dementia (Brooker et al., 2011). Observational methods capture the social interaction of people with dementia, many of whom continue to contribute to the wellbeing of others in the wider community (Hubbard et al., 2003). Dawn Brooker has been instrumental in developing a number of tools that ensure the experience of the person with dementia is recognised in a number of contexts (Brooker et al., 2011).

Summary

- Developing outcome measures that reflect the experience of older people, their families and staff may be problematic as different people want different things from their care experience
- Measures that are developed or used need to reflect what is being measured
- Different tools may suit different contexts and so we need to avoid a 'one size fits all' approach
- Using different data sources rather than relying on one questionnaire might be more helpful in capturing the patient experience
- It may also be useful to assess structural issues such as leadership and teamwork to see how staff are being supported to achieve the outcomes being measured

Table 10.1   Capturing the personal experience by promoting relationships in care environments (PRiCE)

Capturing the personal experience through PRiCE	Not at all	Not often	This does not interest me	Most of the time	Always
Care happens when I/my loved one need it to					
I have confidence in the people supporting me					
I have confidence that the care will be delivered when I /my loved one need it to be					
Important details in my care/ of my loved one are acted upon					
People have time to speak with me					
People who support me know who I am					
People who support me know what matters to me					
People do as they say they will					
I am involved in activities that have meaning for me					
I enjoy having a laugh					
I can have a laugh with those around me					
I feel comfortable here					
I feel comfortable with the support I receive					
I am involved in decisions about things that matter to me					
I make a contribution here					
My contribution is valued					

Conclusion

We have seen throughout this book that participation in the decision-making process enhances the experience of older people, families and staff. Leadership and teamwork are key factors in ensuring a positive experience for older people and their families across care environments. Leadership and teamwork are rarely included in quality evaluations but would capture the role of the organisation in ensuring person-centred and relationship-centred approaches are enabled within the care environment. Examining elements of the biographical assessment and how these are reflected in care records could be incorporated into the quality improvement process through audit. When implementing person-centred and relationship-centred approaches to care, we also need to ensure we are using relevant outcomes such as 'care that matters to me' and/or 'care that involves us all' within the quality process. Capturing the contribution of older people and families is more problematic and may require additional questionnaires and/or observations to ensure all perspectives are represented in the process. We need to be sure that any measures used reflect the appropriate concept and that the concept being measured (such as 'care that matters to me') is understood by all parties. Equally, measures need to be tailored to both the care environment and population of older people whose experience we are interested in.

Note

Information on Care Cards at Inspiration North West. Available at: www.inspirationnw. co.uk/care-cards/

References

Abrahams, A. (2011) *Care and Compassion*? Report of the Health Service Ombudsman on Ten Investigations into NHS Care of Older People. London: Stationery Office.

Age Concern (2006) *Hungry to be Heard: The Scandal of Malnourished Older People in Hospital*. The 'Hungry to be Heard' Report. London: Age Concern England.

Alexander, G., Rantz, M.J., Skubic, M., Koopman, R., Phillips, L., Guevara, R. and Miller, S. (2011) 'Evolution of an early illness warning system to monitor frail elders in independent living', *Journal of Healthcare Engineering*, 2, 259–86.

Anderson, R.A., Issel, L.M. and McDaniel, R.R. Jr. (2003) 'Nursing homes as complex adaptive systems: relationship between management practice and resident outcomes', *Nursing Research*, 52 (1), 12–21.

Anderson, R.A., Ammarell, N., Bailey, D. Jr., Colón-Emeric, C., Corazzini, K.N., Lillie, M., Piven, M.L., Utley-Smith, Q. and McDaniel, R.R. Jr. (2005) 'Nursing assistant mental models, sense making, care actions, and consequences for nursing home residents', *Qualitative Health Research*, 15 (8): 1006–21.

Andrews, G.J., Cutchin, M., McCracken, K., Phillips, D.R. and Wiles, J.L. (2007) 'Geographical gerontology: the constitution of a discipline', *Social Science and Medicine*, 65, 151–68.

Badger, F., Clifford, C., Hewison, A. and Thomas, K. (2009) 'An evaluation of the implementation of a programme to improve end-of-life care in nursing homes', *Palliative Medicine*, 23 (6): 502–11.

Bayer, T., Tadd, W. and Krajcik, S. (2005) 'Dignity: the voice of older people', *Quality in Ageing*, 6 (1): 22–9.

Baylis, J. and Sly, F. (2010) *Ageing Across the UK, Regional Trends 42*. Newport, Wales: Office for National Statistics. Available at: www.ons.gov.uk/ons/publications/index.html (accessed 2 January 2012).

Beach, M.C. and Inui, T. and Relationship Centred Care Network (2006) 'Relationship centred care: a constructive reframing', *Journal of General Internal Medicine*, 21: S3–8.

Booth, J., Kumlien, S. and Zhang, Y. (2009) 'Promoting urinary continence for older people: key issues for nurses, *International Journal of Older People's Nursing*, 4 (1): 63–9.

Bowers, B.J., Esmond, S. and Jacobson, N. (2000) 'The relationship between staffing and quality in long-term care facilities: exploring the views of nurse aides', *Journal of Nursing Care Quality*, 14 (4): 55–64.

Bowers, B.J., Fibich, B. and Jacobson, N. (2001a) 'Practice concepts. Care-as-service, care-as-relating, care-as-comfort: understanding nursing home residents' definitions of quality', *Gerontologist*, 41 (4): 539–45.

Bowers, B.J., Lauring, C. and Jacobson, N. (2001b) 'How nurses manage time and work in long-term care', *Journal of Advanced Nursing*, 33 (4): 484–91.

Bradbury-Jones, C., Irvine, F., Jones, C., Kakehashi, C. and Ogi, A. (2011) 'A comparison of elderly care nursing in the UK and Japan', *Nursing Older People*, 23 (9): 31–5.

Bridges, J., Flatley, M., Meyer, J. and Brown Wilson, C. (2009) *Best Practice for Older People in Acute Care Settings (BPOP): Guidance for Nurses*. Available at: http://nursingstandard.rcnpublishing.co.uk/shared/media/multimedia/index.htm (accessed 26 June 2012).

Bridges, J., Flatley, M. and Meyer, J. (2010) 'Older people's and relatives' experiences in acute care settings: systematic review and synthesis of qualitative studies', *International Journal of Nursing Studies*, 47: 89–107.

Brooker, D. (2004) 'What is person centred care in dementia?', *Reviews in Clinical Gerontology*, 13: 215–22.

Brooker, D., La Fontaine, J., De Vries, K., Porter, T. and Surr, C. (2011) *How Can I Tell You What's Going on Here?* The development of PIECE-dem: an observational framework focusing on the perspective of residents with advanced dementia living in care homes. Association for Dementia Studies, University of Worcester. Available at: http://ihsc.worc.ac.uk/dementia/PIECE-dem%20Final%20report%20June%202011.pdf (accessed 22 June 2012).

Brown, J., Nolan, M., Davies, S., Nolan, J. and Keady, J. (2008) 'Transforming students' views of gerontological nursing: realising the potential of "enriched" environments of learning and care: a multi-method longitudinal study', *International Journal of Nursing Studies*, 45: 1214–32.

Brown Wilson, C.R. (2007) Exploring Relationships in Care Homes: A Constructivist Inquiry. PhD dissertation. University of Sheffield, Sheffield.

Brown Wilson, C. (2009) 'Developing community in care homes through a relationship-centred approach', *Health and Social Care in the Community*, 17 (2): 177–86.

Brown Wilson, C. (2011) 'Working together: policy and older people', in Reed, J., Clarke, C. and McFarlane, A. (eds), *Nursing Older People: A Textbook for Nurses*. Buckingham: Open University Press.

Brown Wilson, C. and Davies, S. (2009) 'Using relationships in care homes to develop relationship centred care: the contribution of staff', *Journal of Clinical Nursing*, 18: 1746–55.

Brown Wilson, C., Cook, G. and Forte, D. (2009a) 'The use of narrative in developing relationships in care homes', in Froggatt, K., Davies, S. and Meyer, J. (eds), *Understanding Care Homes: A Research and Development Perspective*. London: Jessica Kingsley, pp. 70–90.

Brown Wilson, C., Davies, S. and Nolan, M.R. (2009b) 'Developing relationships in care homes: the contribution of staff, residents and families', *Ageing and Society*, 29 (7): 1041–63.

Brown Wilson, C., Tetley, J., Healey, J. and Wolton, R. (2011) 'The best care is like sunshine: creative writing and older people in residential long term care', *Activities, Adaptation and Aging*, 35 (1): 1–20.

Brown Wilson, C., Swarbrick, C., Pilling, M. and Keady, J. (2012) 'The senses in practice: enhancing the quality of care for residents with dementia in care homes', *Journal of Advanced Nursing*.

Carbonneau, H., Caron, C. and Desrosiers, J. (2010) 'Development of a conceptual framework of positive aspects of caregiving in dementia', *Dementia*, 9: 327–53.

Care Quality Commission (CQC) (2010) *Guidance about Compliance: Essential Standards of Quality and Safety*. Available at: www.cqc.org.uk/oranisations-we-regulate (accessed 22 June 2012).

Caron, C.D., Griffith, J. and Arcand, M. (2005) 'End-of-life decision making in dementia: how family caregivers perceive their interactions with health care providers in long-term-care settings', *Journal of Applied Gerontology*, 24: 231–47.

Chao, S.Y., Lan, Y.H., Tso, H.C., Chung, C.M., Neim, Y.M. and Clark, M.J. (2008) 'Predictors of psychosocial adaptation among elderly residents in long-term care settings', *Journal of Nursing Research*, 16 (2): 149–59.

Cheek, J., Ballantyne, A., Byers, L., and Quan, J. (2007) 'From retirement village to residential aged care: what older people and their families say', *Health and Social Care in the Community*, 15 (1): 8–17.

Clarke, A. (2000) 'Using biography to enhance the nursing care of older people', *British Journal of Nursing*, 9(7): 429–33.

Clarke, A., Hanson, E.J. and Ross, H. (2003) 'Seeing the person behind the patient: enhancing the care of older people using a biographical approach', *Journal of Clinical Nursing*, 12: 697.

Clarke, C. and Warren, L. (2007) 'Hopes, fears and expectations about the future: what do older people's stories tell us about active ageing?', *Ageing and Society*, 27: 465–88.

Clissett, P. (2007) A Constructivist Investigation into Relationships Between Community Dwelling Older People and Their Carers. PhD dissertation. University of Sheffield.

Connolly, M., Grimshaw, J., Dodd, M., Cawthorne, J., Hulme, T., Everitt, S., Tierney, S. and Deaton, C. (2009) 'Systems and people under pressure: the discharge process in an acute hospital', *Journal of Clinical Nursing*, 18: 549–58.

Cook, G. and Brown Wilson, C. (2010) 'Care home residents' experiences of social relationships with staff', *Nursing Older People*, 22 (1): 24–9.

Cook, G., Brown Wilson, C. and Forte, D. (2006) 'The impact of sensory impairment on social interaction between residents in care homes', *International Journal of Older People's Nursing*, 1: 216–24.

Cookman, C. (2005) 'Attachment in older adulthood: concept clarification', *Journal of Advanced Nursing*, 50 (5): 528–35.

Corazzini, K., McConnell, E.S., Rapp, C.G. and Anderson, R.A. (2004) 'A conceptual framework for understanding the decision-making processes of nursing assistants in providing dementia care', *Alzheimer's Care Quarterly*, 5 (3): 197–206.

Cornwell, B. (2011) 'Age trends in daily social contact patterns', *Research on Aging*, 33: 598–631.

Coughlan, R. and Ward, L. (2007) 'Experiences of recently relocated residents of a long-term care facility in Ontario: assessing quality qualitatively', *International Journal of Nursing Studies*, 44 (1): 47–57.

Davies, S. and Nolan, M. (2004) '"Making the move": relatives' experiences of the transition to a care home', *Health and Social Care in the Community*, 12 (6): 517–26.

Department of Health (DH) (2000) *National Service Framework for Older People*. Available at: www.doh.gov.uk/nsf/pdfs/nsfolderpeople.pdf (accessed 22 June 2012).

Department of Health (DH) (2003) *Discharge from Hospital: Pathway, Process and Practice*. London: Department of Health.

Department of Health (DH) (2008) *End of Life Care Strategy: Promoting High Quality Care for all Adults at the End of Life*. London: Department of Health/Stationery Office.

Department of Health (DH) (2009) *The Delayed Discharges (Continuing Care) Directions 2009*. London: Department of Health. Available at: www.dh.gov.uk/en/Publicationsandstatistics/Publications/PublicationsLegislation/DH_106178 (accessed 16 April 2012).

Department of Health (DH) (2010) *Ready to Go: Planning the Discharge and Transfer of Patients from Hospital and Intermediate Care*. London: Department of Health. Available at: www.dh.gov.uk/en/Publicationsandstatistics/Publications/PublicationsPolicyAndGuidance/DH_103146 (accessed 16 April 2012).

Dew, C. (2011) *Provisional Monthly HES Data for Admitted Patient Care*. Available at: www.hesonline.nhs.uk/Ease/ContentServer?siteID=1937&categoryID=202 (accessed 2 January 2012).

Dewar, B. (2011) Caring about Caring: An Appreciative Inquiry about Compassionate Relationship-Centred Care. Unpublished PhD thesis. Edinburgh Napier University, Edinburgh. Available at: http://researchrepository.napier.ac.uk/4845/1/PHDFINALBDEWAR2011[1].pdf (accessed 6 January 2012).

Doherty-King, B. and Bowers, B. (2011) 'How nurses decide to ambulate hospitalized older adults: development of a conceptual model', *The Gerontologist*, 51 (6): 786–97.

Donabedian, A. (1966) 'Evaluating the quality of medical care', *Milbank Memorial Fund Quarterly*, 44 (3): 166–203.

Donabedian, A. (1988) 'The quality of care: how can it be assessed?', *Journal of the American Medical Association*, 260 (12): 1743–8.

Elia, M. and Russell, C. (eds) (2007) *Nutrition Screening Survey and Audit of Adults on Admission to Hospitals, Care Homes and Mental Health Units*. British Association for Parenteral and Enteral Nutrition (BAPEN). Available at: www.bapen.org.uk/pdfs/nsw/nsw07_report.pdf (accessed 22 June 2012).

Elia, M. and Russell, C. (eds) (2009) *Combating Malnutrition: Recommendations for Action*. British Association for Parenteral and Enteral Nutrition (BAPEN). Available at: www.bapen. org.uk/professionals/publications-and-resources/bapen-reports/combating-malnutrition-recommendations-for-action (accessed 22 June 2012).

Faulkner, M., Davies, S., Nolan, M.R. and Brown-Wilson, C. (2006) 'Development of the combined assessment of residential environments (CARE) profiles', *Journal of Advanced Nursing*, 55 (6): 664–77.

Ferrucci, L., Guralnik, J.M., Studenski, S., Fried, L.P., Cutler, G.B. and Walston, J.D. (2004) 'Interventions on frailty working group. Designing randomized, controlled trials aimed at preventing or delaying functional decline and disability in frail, older persons: a consensus report', *Journal of the American Geriatric Society*, 52: 625–34.

Flesner, M.K. and Rantz, M.J. (2004) 'Mutual empowerment and respect: effect on nursing home quality of care', *Journal of Nursing Care Quality*, 19 (3): 193–6.

Froggatt, K., Vaughan, S., Bernard, C. and Wild, D. (2009) 'Advance care planning in care homes for older people: an English perspective', *Palliative Medicine*, 23: 332–8.

Funk, L.I., Stajduhar, K., Toye, C., Aoun, S., Grande, G.E. and Todd, C.J. (2010) 'Part 2. Home-based family caregiving at the end of life: a comprehensive review of published qualitative research (1998–2008)', *Palliative Medicine*, 24: 594–607.

Gilliard, J. and Marshall, M. (eds) (2012) *Transforming the Quality of Life for People with Dementia Through Contact with the Natural World*. London: Jessica Kingsley.

Godfrey, M., Townsend, J. and Denby, T. (2004) Building a good life for older people in local communities. The experience of ageing in time and place. Joseph Rowntree Foundation. Available at: www.jrf.org.uk/sites/files/jrf/1859352359.pdf (accessed 22 June 2012).

Goffman, E. (1962) *Asylums: Essays on the Social Situation of Mental Patients and Other Inmates*: Chicago, IL: Aldine.

Goldsmith, M. (2011) 'They maintained the fabric of this world: spirituality and the non-religious', in Jewell, A. (ed.), *Spirituality and Personhood in Dementia*. London: Jessica Kingsley, pp. 165–74.

Goldsmith, M. (2012) 'Dementia, spirituality and nature', in Gilliard, J. and Marshall, M. (eds), *Transforming the Quality of Life for People with Dementia Through Contact with the Natural World*. London: Jessica Kingsley, pp. 17–22.

Goodman, C., Evans, C., Wilcock, J., Froggatt, K., Drennan, V., Sampson, E., Blanchard, M., Bissett, M. and Iliffe, S. (2010) 'End of life care for community dwelling older people with dementia: an integrated review', *International Journal of Geriatric Psychiatry*, 25: 329–37.

Goodrich, J. and Cornwell, J. (2008) *Seeing the Person in the Patient: The Point of Care Review Paper*. London: King's Fund.

Gott, M. (2005) *Sexuality, Sexual Health and Ageing*. Maidenhead: Open University Press.

Gott, M. and Hinchcliffe, S. (2003) 'How important is sex in later life, the views of older people', *Social Science and Medicine*, 56: 1617–28.

Griffiths, P., Jones, S., Maben, J. and Murrells, T. (2008) *State of the Art Metrics for Nursing: A Rapid Appraisal*. London: National Nursing Research Unit, King's College.

Gruneir, A., Silver, M. and Rochon, P. (2011) 'Review. Emergency department use by older adults: a literature review on trends, appropriateness, and consequences of unmet health care needs', *Medical Care Research and Review*, 68: 131–55.

Hall, S., Kolliakou, A., Petkova, H., Froggatt, K. and Higginson, I.J. (2011) 'Interventions for improving palliative care for older people living in nursing care homes', *Cochrane Database of Systematic Reviews*, 3: CD007132.

Hartikainen, S., Lonnroos, E. and Louhivuori, K. (2007) 'Medication as a risk factor for falls: critical systematic review', *Journals of Gerontology. Series A, Biological Sciences and Medical Sciences*, 62 (10): 1172–81.

Hubbard, G., Tester, S. and Downs, M. (2003) 'Meaningful social interactions between older people in institutional care settings', *Ageing and Society*, 23: 99–114.

Hughes, J., Bamford, C. and May, C. (2008) 'Types of centredness in health care: themes and concepts', *Medical Health Care and Philosophy*, 11: 455–63.

Inouye, S., Studenski, S., Tinetti, M. and Kuchel, G. (2007) 'Geriatric syndromes: clinical research and policy implications of a core geriatric concept', *Journal of the American Geriatrics Society*, 55: 780–91.

Institute of Medicine (IoM) (2001) *Crossing the Quality Chasm: A New Health System for the 21st Century*. Washington, DC: National Academy Press.

Iwarsson, S., Wahl, H.W., Nygren, C., Oswald, F., Sixsmith, A., Sixsmith, J., Szé´man, Z. and Tomsone, S. (2007) 'Importance of the home environment for healthy aging: conceptual and methodological background of the European ENABLE-AGE project', *The Gerontologist*, 47 (1): 78–84.

Jacelon, C. (2003) 'The dignity of elders in acute care hospital', *Qualitative Health Research*, 13 (4): 543–56.

Kelsey, S., Laditka, S. and Laditka, J. (2010) 'Caregiver perspectives on transitions to assisted living and memory care', *American Journal of Alzheimer's Disease and Other Dementias*, 25: 255–64.

Kitwood, T. (1997) *Dementia Reconsidered: The Person Comes First*. Buckingham: Open University Press.

Kubrak, C. and Jensen, L. (2007) 'Malnutrition in acute care patients: a narrative review', *International Journal of Nursing Studies*, 44: 1036–54.

Lawrence, V., Samsi, K., Murray, J., Harari, D. and Banerjee, S. (2011) 'Dying well with dementia: qualitative examination of end-of-life care', *The British Journal of Psychiatry* 199 (5): 417–22.

Lee, R. and Mason, A. (2011) *The Generational Economy: A Global Perspective*. Northampton, MA: Edward Elgar for International Development Research Centre.

Levenson, R. (2007) *The Challenge of Dignity in Care: Upholding the Rights of the Individual*. London: Help the Aged.

Lutz, B.J. and Bowers, B.J. (2000) 'Patient-centred care: understanding its interpretation and implementation in health care', *Scholarly Inquiry for Nursing Practice: An International Journal*, 14 (2): 165–82.

Mapes, N. (2012) 'Living with dementia through the changing seasons', in Gilleard, J. and Marshall, M. (eds), *Transforming the Quality of Life for People with Dementia Through Contact with the Natural World*. London: Jessica Kingsley, pp. 30–43.

McAuliffe, L., Nay, R. and Bauer, M. (2012) 'Sexuality and intimacy', in Reed, J., Clarke, C. and McFarlane, A. (eds), *Nurisng Older Adults*. Maidenhead: Open University Press, pp. 191–203.

McClelland, T. (2007) *Protected Meal Times*. Available at: www.rcn.org.uk/_data/assets/word_doc/0019/69031/Protected_Mealtimes.doc (accessed 4 September 2011).

McCormack, B. (2004) 'Person-centredness in gerontological nursing: an overview of the literature', *International Journal of Older People Nursing* in association with *Journal of Clinical Nursing*, 13 (3a): 31–38.

McCormack, B. and McCance, T. (2006) 'Development of a framework for person centred nursing', *Journal of Advanced Nursing*, 56 (5): 472–9.

McCormack, B. and McCance, T. (2010) *Person Centred Nursing: Theory and Practice*. Oxford: Wiley Blackwell.

McKeown, J., Clarke, A. and Repper, J. (2006) 'Life story work in health and social care: systematic literature review', *Journal of Advanced Nursing*, 55 (2): 237–47.

McNair, D. (2012) 'Sunlight and daylight', in Gilliard, J. and Marshall, M. (eds), *Transforming the Quality of Life for People with Dementia Through Contact with the Natural World*. London: Jessica Kingsley, pp. 23–9.

Mead, N. and Bower, P. (2000) 'Patient-centredness: a conceptual framework and review of the empirical literature', *Social Science and Medicine*, 51: 1087–110.

Milisen, K., Lemiengre, J., Braes, T. and Foreman, M. (2005) 'Multicomponent intervention strategies for managing delirium in hospitalized older people: systematic review', *Journal of Advanced Nursing*, 52 (1): 79–90.

Minkler, M. (1996) 'Critical perspectives on ageing: new challenges for gerontology', *Ageing and Society*, 16: 467–87.

Molony, L., Evans, L., Jeon, S., Rabig, J. and Straka, L. (2011) 'Trajectories of at-homeness and health in usual care and small house nursing homes', *The Gerontologist*, 51 (4): 504–15.

Moos, I. and Bjorn, A. (2006) 'Use of the life story in the institutional care of people with dementia: a review of intervention studies', *Ageing and Society*, 26: 431–54.

Mowatt, H. (2011) 'Voicing the spiritual: working with people with dementia', in Jewell, A. (ed.), *Spirituality and Personhood in Dementia*. London: Jessica Kingsley, pp. 75–86.

Nakrem, S., Guttormsen Vinsnes, A., Harkless, G., Paulsen, B. and Seim, A. (2009) 'Nursing sensitive quality indicators for nursing home care: international review of literature, policy and practice', *International Journal of Nursing Studies*, 46: 848–57.

National Collaborating Centre for Nursing and Supportive Care (2004) *Clinical Practice Guideline for the Assessment and Prevention of Falls in Older People (full NICE guideline)*. Clinical guideline 21. London: Royal College of Nursing. Available at: www.nice.org.uk (accessed 26 January 2009).

National Health Service (NHS) Information (2012) *Provisional Monthly Patient Reported Outcome Measures (PROMs) in England – April 2011 to January 2012: Pre- and Post-operative Data*. Available at: http://www.ic.nhs.uk/pubs/provisionalmonthlyproms (accessed 22 June 2012).

National Institute for Health and Clinical Excellence (NICE) (2006) *Nutrition Support in Adults: Oral Nutrition Support, Enteral Tube Feeding and Parenteral Nutrition*. Clinical guideline 32. London: National Institute for Health and Clinical Excellence.

National Patient Safety Agency (2009) *Protected Mealtimes Review: Findings and Recommendations Report*. London: National Patient Safety Agency.

Nieuwenhuizen, W., Weenen, H., Rigby, P. and Hetherington, M. (2010) 'Older adults and patients in need of nutritional support: review of current treatment options and factors influencing nutritional intake', *Clinical Nutrition*, 29 (2): 160–9.

Nolan, M.R., Brown, J., Davies, S., Nolan, J. and Keady, J. (2006) *The Senses Framework: Improving Care for Older People Through a Relationship Centred Approach*. GRip Report. University of Sheffield.

Nolan, M.R., Davies, S., Brown, J., Keady, J. and Nolan, J. (2004) 'Beyond "person-centred" care: a new vision for gerontological nursing', *International Journal of Older People Nursing* in association with *Journal of Clinical Nursing*, 13 (3a): 45–53.

Nolan, M.R., Grant, G. and Keady, J. (1996) *Understanding Family Care*. Buckingham: Open University Press.

Norris, E., Shelton, F. and Marion, M. (2011) 'Hetherington/ e-SPEN', *European e-Journal of Clinical Nutrition and Metabolism*, 6: e106–e8.

Nygren, C., Oswald, F., Iwarsson, S., Fänge, A., Sixsmith, J., Schilling, O., Sixsmith, A., Széman, Z., Tomsone, S. and Wahl, H.W. (2007) 'Relationships between objective and perceived housing in very old age', *The Gerontologist*, 47 (1): 85–95.

Orpwood, R., Bjørneby, S., Hagen, I., Mäki, O., Faulkner, R. and Topo, P. (2004) 'User involvement in dementia product development', *Dementia*, 3: 263–79.

Oswald, F., Jopp, D., Rott, C. and Wahl, H.W. (2010) 'Is aging in place a resource for or risk to life satisfaction?', *The Gerontologist*, 51 (2): 238–50.

Oswald, F., Wahl, H.W., Schilling, O., Nygren, C., Fänge, A., Sixsmith, A., Sixsmith, J., Széman, Z., Tomsone, S. and Iwarsson, S. (2007) 'Relationships between housing and healthy aging in very old age', *The Gerontologist*, 47 (1): 96–107.

Parker, D. and Froggatt, K. (2011) "Palliative care with older people', in Tolson, D., Booth, J. and Schofield, I. (eds), *Evidence Informed Nursing with Older People*. Oxford: Wiley Blackwell, pp. 84–100.

Patmore, C. and McNulty, A. (2005) *Making Home Care for Older People More Flexible and Person Centred: Factors which Promote This*. York: University of York, Social Policy Research Unit. Available at: www.york.ac.uk/inst/spru/pubs/rworks/aug2005.pdf (accessed 30 January 2007).

Patterson, M., Nolan, M., Rick, J., Brown, J., Adams, R. and Musson, G. (2011) *From Metrics to Meaning: Culture Change and Quality of Acute Hospital Care for Older People*. Final Report: SDO Project (08/1501/93). Available at: www.sdo.nihr.ac.uk/projlisting. php?cat=completed&ord=invea (accessed 15 March 2011).

Peace, S., Holland, C. and Kellaher, L. (2011) '"Option recognition" in later life: variations in ageing in place', *Ageing and Society*, 31 (5): 734–57.

Philp, I. (2006) *A New Ambition for Old Age*. London: Department of Health.

Powers, B.A. (1991) 'The meaning of nursing home friendships', *Advances in Nursing Science*, 14 (2): 42–58.

Quinn, C., Clare, L. and Woods, B. (2009) 'The impact of the quality of relationship on the experiences and wellbeing of caregivers of people with dementia: a systematic review', *Aging and Mental Health*, 13 (2): 143–54.

Rantz, M.J. and Zwygart-Stauffacher, M. (2004) 'Back to the fundamentals of care: a roadmap to improve nursing home care quality', *Journal of Nursing Care Quality*, 19 (2): 92–4.

Rantz, M.J., Marek, K.D., Aud, M.A., Tyrer, H.W., Skubic, M., Demiris, G. and Hussam, A.A. (2005) 'Technology and nursing collaboration to help older adults age in place', *Nursing Outlook*, 53 (1): 40–5.

Rantz, M.J., Skubic, M., Alexander, G., Aud, M., Wakefield, B., Galambos, J., Koopman, R. and Miller, S. (2010) 'Improving nurse care coordination with technology', *Cin-Computers Informatics Nursing*, 28: 325–32.

Rantz, M.J., Skubic, M., Koopman, R., Phillips, L., Alexander, G., Miller, S. and Guevara, R. (2011) *Using Sensor Networks to Detect Urinary Tract Infections in Older Adults*.

Proceedings of the 13th IEEE International Conference on E-Health Networking and Applications. PID1858641.

Reed, J., Cook, G., Sullivan, A. and Burridge, C. (2003) 'Making a move: care-home residents' experience of relocation', *Ageing and Society*, 23: 225–41.

Risjord, M. (2009) 'Rethinking concept analysis', *Journal of Advanced Nursing*, 65 (3): 684–91.

Robinson, L., Hutchings, D., Corner, L., Beyer, F., Dickinson, H., Vanoli, A., Finch, T., Hughes, J., Ballard, C., May, C. and Bond, J. (2006) 'A systematic literature review of the effectiveness of non-pharmacological interventions to prevent wandering in dementia and evaluation of the ethical implications and acceptability of their use', *Health Technology Assessment*, 10 (26): iii, ix–108.

Rockwood, K., Mitnitski, A., Song, X., Steen, B. and Skoog, I. (2006) 'Long-term risks of death and institutionalization of elderly people in relation to deficit accumulation at age 70', *Journal of the American Geriatric Society*, 54 (6): 975–9.

Rolls, L., Seymour, J., Froggatt, K.A. and Hanratt, B. (2011) 'Older people living alone at the end of life in the UK: research and policy challenges', *Palliative Medicine*, 25: 650–7.

Ronch, J. (2004) 'Changing institutional culture: can we re-value the nursing home?', *Journal of Gerontological Social Work*, 43 (1): 61–82.

Roper, N., Logan W. and Tierney, A. (2001) *The Roper–Logan–Tierney Model of Nursing: Based on Activities of Living*. London: Churchill-Livingstone.

Rossen, E. and Knafl, K. (2003) 'Older women's response to residential relocation: description of transition styles', *Qualitative Health Research*, 13: 20–36.

Royal College of Nursing (2007) *Water for Health Hydration: Best Practice Toolkit for Hospitals and Healthcare*. Water UK. London: Royal College of Nursing. Available at: www.rcn.org.uk/_data/assets/pdf_file/0004/70375/Hydration_Toolkit_-_cover.pdf (accessed 16 April 2012).

Ryan, T., Nolan, M.R., Reid, D. and Enderby, P. (2008) 'Using the senses framework to achieve relationship-centred dementia care services: a case example', *Dementia: The International Journal of Social Research and Practice*, 7 (1): 71–93.

Schneider, J., Scales, K., Bailey, S. and Lloyd, J. (2010) *Challenging Care: The Role and Experience of Health Care Assistants in Dementia Wards*. SDO project 1819/222. Available at: www.panicoa.org.uk/panicoa-studies/challenging-care-role-and-experience-health-care-assistants-dementia-wards (accessed 3 January 2012).

Seymour, J., Kumar, A. and Froggatt, K. (2011) 'Do nursing homes for older people have the support they need to provide end-of-life care? A mixed methods enquiry in England', *Palliative Medicine*, 25: 125–38.

Shippee, T.P. (2009) 'But I am not moving: residents' perspectives on transitions within a continuing care retirement community', *The Gerontologist*, 49 (3): 418–27.

Siddiqui, N., Holt, R., Britton, A.M. and Holmes, J. (2007) 'Interventions for preventing delirium in hospitalised patients', *Cochrane Database of Systematic Reviews*, 2: CD005563.

Simmons, S., Rahman, A., Beuscher, L., Jani, V., Durkin, D. and Schnelle, J. (2011) 'Resident-directed long-term care: staff provision of choice during morning care', *The Gerontologist*, 51 (6): 867–75.

Skelton, D., Dinan, S., Campbell, M. and Rutherford, O. (2005) 'Frequent fallers halve the risk of falls within 9 months of tailored group exercise (FaME): an RCT in community dwelling women aged 65 and over', *Age and Ageing*, 34: 636–9.

Skelton, D., McAloon, M. and Gray, L. (2011) 'Promoting physical activity with older people', in Tolson, D., Booth, J. and Schofield, I. (eds), *Evidence Informed Nursing with Older People*. Oxford: Blackwell.

Stajduhar, K.I., Funk, L., Toye, C., Grande, G.E., Aoun, S. and Todd, C.J. (2010) 'Part 1. Home-based family caregiving at the end of life: a comprehensive review of published quantitative research (1998–2008)', *Palliative Medicine*, 24: 573–93.

Stephens, C., Alpass, F., Towers, A. and Stevenson, B. (2011) 'The effects of types of social networks, perceived social support and loneliness on the health of older people: accounting for the social context', *Journal of Aging and Health*, 23 (6): 887–911.

Tadd, W., Hillman, A., Calnan, S., Calnan, M., Bayer, T. and Read, S. (2011) *Dignity in Practice: An Exploration of the Care of Older Adults in Acute NHS Trusts*. Service Delivery and Organisation Programme. Available at: www.sdo.nihr.ac.uk/files/project/SDO_FR_08-1819-218_V01.pdf (accessed 16 April 2012).

Thein, N-W., D'Souza, G. and Sheehan, B. (2011) 'Expectations and experience of moving to a care home: perceptions of older people with dementia', *Dementia*, 10(1): 7–18.

Thomas, L.H., Cross, S., Barrett, J., French, B., Leathley, M., Sutton, C.J., Watkins, C. (2008) 'Treatment of urinary incontinence after stroke in adults', *Cochrane Database of Systematic Reviews*, Iss. 1. Art. No.: CD004462. DOI: 10.1002/14651858.CD004462. pub3.

Thompson and Sheth, Patient Satisfaction Coventry University (2008) Available at: www. patientexperiencefeedback.com/measuring_patient_satisfaction/coventry_university_research.html (accessed 16 August 2012).

Tolson, D. and Brown Wilson, C (2011) 'Communication', in J. Reed, C. Clarke and A. McFarlane (eds) *Nursing Older People: A Textbook for Nurses*. Buckingham: Open University Press.

Tolson, D., Day, T. and Booth, J. (2011) 'Age related hearing problems', in Tolson, D., Booth, J. and Schofield, I. (eds), *Evidence Informed Nursing with Older People*. Oxford: Blackwell.

Torrington, J. (2007) 'Evaluating quality of life in residential care buildings', *Building Research and Information*, 35 (5): 514–28.

Townsend, P. (1962) *The Last Refuge: A Survey of Residential Institutions and Homes for the Aged in England and Wales*. London: Routledge and Kegan Paul.

Tresolini, C.P. and the Pew-Fetzer Task Force (1994) *Health Professions Education and Relationship-Centred Care*. San Francisco, CA: Pew Health Professions Commission.

Turner, D., Little, P., Raftery, J., Turner, S., Smith, H., Rumsby, K. and Mullee, M. (2010) 'Cost effectiveness of management strategies for urinary tract infections: results from randomised controlled trial', *British Medical Journal*, 340: c346. Available at: www.bmj. com/content/340/bmj.c346.full (accessed 16 August 2012).

Wadensten, B. (2005) 'The content of morning time conversations between nursing home staff and residents', *Journal of Clinical Nursing*, 14 (s2): 84–9.

Ward, R., Vaas, A., Aggarwal, N., Cybyk, B. and Garfield, C. (2005) 'A kiss is still a kiss? The construction of sexuality in dementia care', *Dementia*, 4: 49–72.

Wenger, G.C. and Tucker, I. (2002) 'Using network variation in practice: identification of support network type', *Health and Social Care in the Community*, 10 (1): 28–35.

Wilde, B., Larsonn, G. et al. (1995) 'Quality of care from the elderly person's perspective: subjective importance and perceived reality', *Ageing Clinical and Experimental Research*, 7:140–9.

Wiles, J. (2005) 'Conceptualising place in the care of older people: the contribution of geographical gerontology', *International Journal of Older People Nursing* in association with *Journal of Clinical Nursing*, 14 (8b): 100–8.

Wiles, J., Leibing, A., Guberman, N., Reeve, J. and Allen, R. (2012) 'The meaning of "ageing in place" to older people', *The Gerontologist*, 52(3): 357–66.

World Health Organization (WHO) (2002) *Ageing: A Policy Framework*. Geneva: World Health Organization. Available at: http://whqlibdoc.who.int/hq/2002/WHO_NMH_ NPH_02.8.pdf (accessed 30 March 2012).

World Health Organization (WHO) (2003) *Definitions of Palliative Care*. Geneva: World Health Organization.

World Health Organization (WHO) (2009) *World Health Statistics 2009*. Geneva: World Health Organization. Available at: www.who.int/whosis/whostat/EN_WHS09_Full.pdf (accessed 30 March 2012).

World Health Organization (WHO) (2010) *Sexual and Reproductive Health: Gender and Human Rights*. Geneva: World Health Organization.

Zeanandin, G., Molato, O., Le Duff, F., Guérin, O., Hébuterne, X. and Schneider, S. (2012) 'Impact of restrictive diets on the risk of undernutrition in a free-living elderly population', *Clinical Nutrition*, 31 (1): 69–73.

Zimmerman, S., Philip, D., Sloane, P., Williams, C., Reed, P., Preisser, J., Eckert, J.K., Boustani, M. and Dobbs, D. (2005) 'Dementia care and quality of life in assisted living and nursing homes', *The Gerontologist*, 45 (Special Issue I): 133–46.

Zisberg, A., Young, H., Scepp, K. and Zysberg, L. (2007) 'A concept analysis of routine: relevance to nursing', *Journal of Advanced Nursing*, 57 (4): 442–53.

Zunzunegui, M.V., Kone, A., Johri, M., Beland, F., Wolfson, C. and Bergman, H. (2004) 'Social networks and self-rated health in two French-speaking Canadian community dwelling populations over 65', *Social Science and Medicine*, 58: 2069–81.

Index

Note: Locators in *italics* refer to tables and figures.